61034

WITHD

OM

WITHDRAWN

61034

OM.

Creative Meditations from Alan Watts

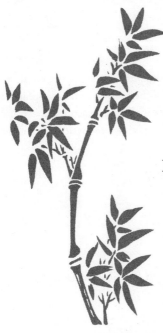

Edited and Adapted by
Judith Johnstone

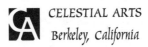

CELESTIAL ARTS
Berkeley, California

These transcripts represent a small selection from the Alan Watts Tape
Archives. For further information on the spoken word of Alan Watts,
write to:

Electronic University
P.O. Box 2309
San Anselmo, California 94979

Copyright © 1980, 1995 by Electronic University

CELESTIAL ARTS
P.O. Box 7123
Berkeley, California 94707

No part of this book may be reproduced by any mechanical, photo-
graphic, or electronic process, or in the form of a phonographic recording, nor may it be stored in a retrieval system, transmitted, or otherwise
be copied for public or private use, without the written permission of
the publisher.

Cover and text design by Toni Tajima.
Cover photo by Pirkle Jones.

First Printing, March, 1980

Library of Congress Cataloging in Publication Data
Watts, Alan Wilson, 1915-1973.
  Om, creative meditations.
  1. Spiritual Life. 2. Meditations. 1. Title.
BL624.W37 1980 191 79-54101
ISBN 0-89087-793-9

8   9   10   11   12   –   99   98   97   96   95

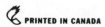 PRINTED IN CANADA

61034

Table of Contents

Foreword

THE FOLLOWING MEDITATIONS were transcribed from lectures which, during many hours of listening, emerged as outstanding examples of my father's teachings. My selections were carefully edited and adapted by Judith Johnstone, who has proven to be eminently equal to the delicate task of transferring spoken words into print. I am delighted to see how successfully the original impact and flavor of these talks has been captured.

As you read through these pages, you will find that the text still contains the easy rhythms of his speech, and you may find it enjoyable to read sections aloud to yourself and to your friends.

Mark Watts
Mill Valley, California
Spring, 1980

Introduction

A person who thinks all the time has nothing to think about except thoughts, so he loses touch with reality and lives in a world of illusions. By thoughts, I mean specifically "chatter in the skull," a perpetual and compulsive repetition of words, of reckoning, and calculating. I am not saying that thinking is bad. Like everything else, it is useful in moderation; a good servant but a bad master. All so-called civilized peoples have increasingly become crazy and self-destructive because, through excessive thinking, they have lost touch with reality. That is to say, we confuse science, words, numbers, symbols, and ideas with the real world. Most of us would rather have money than tangible wealth; a great occasion is somehow spoiled for us unless photographed; and to read about it the next day in the newspaper is oddly more fun for us than the original event. This is a disaster. For, as a result of confusing the real world of nature with mere signs, such as bank balances and contracts, we are destroying nature. We are so tied up in our minds that we have lost our senses, and do not realize that the air stinks, water tastes of chlorine, the human landscape looks like a trash heap, and much of our food tastes like plastic. It is time to wake up.

What is reality? Obviously no one can say, because it is not words. It is not material; that is just an idea. It is not spiritual; that is also an idea, a symbol. We all know what reality is, but we cannot describe it, just as we all know how to beat our hearts and shape our bones, but cannot say how it is done. To get in touch with reality, there is an art of meditation, of what is called yoga or *dhana* in India, *chan* in China, and *zen* in Japan. It is the art of temporarily silencing the mind, of stopping the chatter in the skull. Of course, you cannot force your mind to be silent. That would be like trying to smooth ripples in water with an iron. Water becomes clear and calm only when left alone.

DYANA: The Art of Meditation

The art of meditation is a way of getting in touch with reality. The reason for meditation is that most civilized people are out of touch with reality because they confuse the world as it is with the world as they think about it, talk about it, and describe it. On the one hand, there is the real world and, on the other, a whole system of symbols about that world which we have in our minds. These are very, very useful symbols and all civilization depends on them, but like all good things, they have their disadvantages. The principle disadvantage of symbols is that we confuse them with reality, just as we confuse money with actual wealth, and our images of ourselves with ourselves. Now, of course, "reality" from a philosopher's point of view is a dangerous word. A philosopher will ask, "What do I mean by reality? Am I talking about the physical world of nature, or am I talking about a spiritual world?" To that I have a very simple answer: When we talk about the material world, that is actually a philosophical concept. In the same way, if I say that reality is spiritual, that is also a philosophical concept and reality itself is not a concept. Reality is...and we won't give it a name.

Now, what does not exist in the real world is amazing. For example, in the real world, there are not any things, nor are there any events. That does not mean to say that the real world is a featureless blank. On the contrary, it is a marvelous system of wiggles in which we describe things and events in the same way as we would project images on a Rorschach blot, or pick out particular groups of stars in the sky and call them constellations, as if they were actually separate. Well, they are groups of stars in the mind's eye, in our system of concepts, but they are not "out there" as constellations grouped in the sky. So, in the same way, the difference between myself and all the rest of the universe is nothing more than an idea. It is not a real difference, and meditation is the way in which we come to feel our basic inseparability from the whole universe. Now what that requires is that we shut up. That is to say, we become interiorly silent and cease the interminable chatter that goes on inside our skulls. Most of us think compulsively all the time; that is to say, we talk to ourselves. I remember when I was a boy we had a common saying, "Talking to yourself is the first sign of madness." Obviously, if I talk all the time, I do not hear what anyone else has to say. So, in exactly the same way, if I think all the time, that is to say, if I talk to myself all the time, I do not have anything to think about except thoughts, and live entirely in the world of symbols, and am never in relationship with reality.

That is the first basic reason for meditation, but there is another sense in which we would say that meditation does *not* have a reason or a purpose. In this respect it is unlike almost all other things we do except perhaps playing music and dancing. When we play music we do not do it in order to reach a certain point, such as the end of the composition. If the purpose of music were to get to the end of the piece then the fastest players would be the best. Likewise, when we are dancing, we are not aiming to arrive at a particular place on the floor as we would be if we were taking a journey. When we dance, the journey itself is the point. When we play music, the playing itself is the point, and the same is true of meditation. Meditation is the discovery that the point of life is always arrived at in the immediate moment. Therefore, if you meditate for an ulterior motive, that is to say, to improve your mind, to improve your character, to be more efficient in life, you have your eye on the future and you are not meditating. The future is a concept; it does not exist. As the proverb says, "Tomorrow never comes," because there is no such thing as tomorrow, and there never will be because the time is always now.

That is one of the things we discover when we stop talking to ourselves and stop thinking. We find there is only a present, only an eternal now. It is funny that one meditates for no reason at all except, we could say, for the enjoyment of it. Here I would interpose the essential principle, that meditation is supposed to be fun. It is not something to be done as a grim duty. Indeed, the trouble with religion as we know it is that it is completely mixed up with grim duties. We do it because "it is good for you" and it has become almost a kind of self-punishment. However, meditation, when correctly done, has nothing to do with all that. It is an appreciation of the present, a kind of "grooving" with the eternal now, and it brings us into a state of peace where we can understand that the point of life, the place where it is at, is simply here and now.

In the art of meditation there are various props or supports. One tool that we use as a means of stilling chatter in the mind is pure sound and for that reason it is useful to have a gong. I use a Japanese Buddhist gong made of bronze and shaped like a bowl. If you do not have one of those, you can use the rounded end of a oxygen tank. Simply have a machinist saw it off in the shape of a bowl. You can also simply use your own voice in many kinds of chanting.

Now then, how does one sit in meditation? You may sit any way you want. You may sit in a chair or you may sit on your knees, or in the lotus posture, which is more difficult. The lotus posture is to sit cross-legged with the feet on the thighs, soles upwards. The younger you are when you start, the easier you will find it to do. You can also just sit cross-legged on a raised cushion above the floor. The point of this is that if you keep your back erect, you are centered and easily balanced and you have a feeling of being thoroughly rooted to the ground. That sort of physical stability is very important for avoiding distraction and generally feeling settled. Here and now, as the French say, "Je suis, je reste," "I am here, and I am going to stay."

The easiest way to get into the meditative state is to begin by listening. Simply allow yourself to hear all the sounds that are going on around you. Listen to the general hum and buzz of the world as if you were listening to music. Do not try to identify the sounds you are hearing; do not put names on them. Simply allow them to play within your eardrums and let them go. In other words, let your ears hear whatever they want to hear. Do not judge the sounds. There are no proper sounds or improper sounds, and it does not matter if somebody coughs, sneezes, or drops something. It is all just sound. Do not try to make any sense out of what you are hearing because your brain will take care of that automatically. You do not have to try to understand anything, just listen to the sound. As you pursue that experiment you will very naturally find that you cannot help naming sounds and identifying them. You will go on thinking, that is to say, talking to yourself inside your head, automatically. It is important that you do not try to repress those thoughts by forcing them out of your mind, because that will have precisely the same effect as if you were trying to smooth ripples in water with a flat iron. You are just going to disturb it all the more. As you hear sounds coming up in your head or thoughts, simply listen to them as part of the general noise going on, just as you would be listening to cars going by or to birds chattering outside the window. Look at your own thoughts as just noises, and soon you will find that the "outside world" and the "inside world" come together. They are a happening. Your thoughts are a happening, just like the sounds going on outside, and all you are doing is watching it.

In this process, another thing that is going on is that you are breathing. As you begin meditation, allow your breath to run, just as it will. In other words, do not do a breathing exercise, but just watch your breath breathing the way it wants to breathe. You may notice a curious thing about this. You say in the ordinary way, "I breathe," because you feel that breathing is something that you are doing voluntarily, just in the same way as you might be walking or talking. However, you will also notice that when you are not thinking about breathing, your breathing goes on just the same. The curious thing about breath is that it can be looked at both as a voluntary and an involuntary action. You can feel, on the one hand, "I am doing it," and on the other hand, "It is happening to me." That is why breathing is a most important part of meditation because it is going to show you, as you become aware of your breath, that the hard and fast division that we make between what we do and what happens to us is arbitrary. As you watch your breathing you will become aware that both the voluntary and the involuntary aspects of your experience are all one happening. At first, this may seem a little scary, because you may think, "Well, am I just the puppet of a happening, the mere passive witness of something that is going on completely beyond my control? Or, am I really doing everything that is going along? Of course, that would be very embarrassing, because I would be in charge of everything which is a terribly responsible position." The truth of the matter, as you will see, is that both things are true. You can see that everything is happening to you *and* you are doing everything. For example, it is your eyes that are turning the sun into light. It is the nerve ends in your skin that are turning electric vibrations in the air into heat and temperature. It is your ears that are turning vibrations in the air into sound. In that way, you are creating the world, but when we are not talking or philosophizing about it, then there is just this happening.

When you breathe for a while, just letting it happen and not forcing it in any way, you will discover a curious thing. Without making any effort, you can breathe more and more deeply. In other words, suppose you simply are breathing out the breath of relaxation and heave a sigh of relief; you get the sensation that your breath is falling out. Your breath is dropping, dropping out, with the same sort of feeling you might have if you were settling down into an extremely comfortable bed. You become just as heavy as possible and let yourself go. You let your breath go out in just that way. When it is thoroughly, comfortably out and it feels like coming back again, you pull it back in. Now, let your lungs expand, expand, expand until they feel comfortably full, wait a moment, let it stay there, and then, once again, let it fall out. So, in this way, you will discover that your breath gets quite naturally easier and easier, and slower and slower, and more and more powerful. With these various aids—listening to sound, listening to your own interior feelings and thoughts just as if they were something going on, and watching your breath as a happening that is neither voluntary nor involuntary—you begin to be in the state of meditation. Do not hurry anything. Do not worry about the future. Do not worry about what progress you are making; just be entirely content to be aware of what is. Do not be terribly selective or particular and say, "I should think of this, and not of that." Just watch whatever is happening.

Now, some people might say you are out of your mind to simply watch in this way, but to go out of your mind at least once a day is tremendously important because by doing this you come to your senses. If you stay in your mind all the time, you are overly rational. In other words, you are like a very rigid bridge which, because it has got no give, no craziness in it, is going to be blown down in the first hurricane. A lot of yoga teachers try to get you to control your own mind to prove to you that you cannot do it. There is a saying that "a fool who persists in his folly will become wise." So, what they do is they speed up the folly because when you concentrate you can have a certain amount of superficial and initial success by a process commonly called self-hypnosis. You can think you are making progress, and a good teacher will let you go along that way for a while until he really throws you one: "Why are you concentrating?" The method of Buddhism works in this way. Buddha said, "If you suffer, you suffer because you desire, and your desires are either unattainable or always being disappointed. So cut out desire." Those disciples went away, and they stamped on desire, jumped on desire, cut the throat of desire, and threw out desire. But then they came back and Buddha said, "But you are still desiring not to desire." Then, they wondered how to get rid of that. However, it works like this, and all spiritual discipline works in the same way, because the would-be "catchee" is the catcher. That is like desiring not to desire, loving out of a sense of duty, or trying to be spontaneous because you ought to be. All that is nonsense or what is commonly known as lifting yourself up by your own bootstraps. So, when you see that is nonsense, a quietness naturally comes over you and, in seeing that you cannot control your mind, you realize there is no controller. What you took to be the thinker of thoughts is just one of the thoughts. What you took to be the feeler of the feelings was just one of the feelings. What you took to be the experiencer of experience is just part of the experience.

There is not any thinker of thoughts or feeler of feelings. We get ourselves into this bind because we have a grammatical rule that verbs have to have subjects. The funny thing about this is that verbs are processes and subjects are nouns, which are supposed to be things. Now does a noun start a verb? How does a thing put a process into action? Obviously it cannot, but we always insist that there is a subject called the "knower" and without a knower there cannot be knowing. Remember, however, that it is just a grammatical rule; it is not a rule of nature. In nature there is just knowing and feeling, and it is misleading to say, "you are feeling it," as if you were somehow different from the feeling. When I say, "I am feeling," what I mean is, "there is feeling here." When I say, "You are feeling," I mean, "there is feeling there." That I even have to say, "there is feeling," reveals how cumbersome our language is. Chinese is easier because you do not have to put all that in, and so you can say things twice as fast in Chinese as you can in any other language.

When you come to realize that you can do nothing,

that the play of thought and of feeling just goes on by itself as a happening, you are in a state which we will call meditation and slowly, without being pushed, your thoughts will come to silence. That is to say, all the verbal, symbolic chatter going on in the skull will cease. So do not try and get rid of it, because that will again produce the illusion that there is a controller. It just goes on, it goes on, it goes on and finally it gets tired of itself and bored, and stops. So, then, there is a silence and this is a deeper level of meditation. And in that silence, you suddenly begin to see the world as it is. You do not see any past and you do not see any future. You do not see any difference between yourself and the rest of it. That is just an idea. You cannot put your hand on the difference between myself and you. You cannot blow it, you cannot bounce it, you cannot pull it; it is just an idea. You cannot find any material body because a material body is an idea. So is a spiritual body; these are somebody's philosophical notions. Reality is not material; that is an idea. Reality is not spiritual; that is an idea. So we find that we live in an eternal now. You have all the time in the world because you have all the time there is, which is now, and you are this universe. You may feel strange when ideas do not define the differences and other people's doings are your doings because that makes it very difficult to blame other people. Of course, if you are not sophisticated theologically, you may run screaming in the streets and say that you are God. In a way, that is what happened to Jesus because he was not theologically sophisticated. He had only Old Testament biblical theology as a frame of reference. If he had known Hindu theology, he could have put it more subtly, but he had only that rather primitive theology of the Old Testament with God as the monarchical boss. Of course, you cannot go around and say, "I'm the boss's son." If you are going to say, "I am God," you must allow it for everyone else too, and this was a heretical idea from the point of view of Hebrew theology. So, what they did with Jesus is they placed him on a pedestal. They kicked him upstairs so that he would not be able to influence anyone else. "Only you may be God," they said and that stopped the Gospel cold, right at the beginning, because it could not spread.

This is, therefore, to say that the transformation of human consciousness through meditation is frustrated so long as we think of it in terms of something that I, myself, can bring about by some kind of wangle or gimmick. That leads to endless games of spiritual one-upmanship and guru competitions: "My guru is more effective than your guru." "My yoga is faster than your yoga." "I am more aware of myself than you are." "I am humbler than you are." "I am sorrier for my sins than you are." "I love you more than you love me." There are the interminable goings-on about which people fight, disputing whether they are a little bit more evolved than somebody else. However, all that can just fall away and then we get a strange feeling that we have had in our lives only occasionally.

Some people get a glimpse of the fact that we are no longer this poor little stranger "afraid in a world it never made," but that we are this universe. You are creating it at every moment because it starts now. It did not begin in the past because there was no past. If the universe began in the past, when that happened, it was now. Well, it is still now, and the universe is still beginning now and it is trailing off like the wake of a ship from now. The wake of the ship fades out and so does the past. You can look back there to explain things, but the explanation just disappears. You will never find it there because things are not explained by the past. They are explained by what happens now; that creates the past, and it begins here. That is the birth of responsibility, because otherwise you can always look over your shoulder and say, "Well, I am the way I am because my mother dropped me. And she dropped me because she was neurotic because her mother dropped her." You can go back to Adam and Eve or to disappearing monkeys or some such thing, but you will never get at it. In this way you are faced with the fact that you are doing all this. It is an extraordinary shock. So, cheer up! You cannot blame anyone else for the kind of world you are in, and that helps a great deal because most of the good things we are trying to do are based on blaming somebody else and trying to improve them. "Kindly let me help you or you'll drown," said the monkey putting the fish safely up a tree. If we could stop blaming others it would be very difficult to go to war with a straight face. And if you know that "I" in the sense of the person, the front, the ego, really does not exist, then it will not go to your head too badly if you wake up and discover that you are God.

Who Am I?

What do you mean when you say, "I"?

What do you feel when you say, "myself"?

What you are in your innermost being escapes your examination in much the same way that you cannot look directly into your eyes without using a mirror, you cannot bite your own teeth, and you cannot touch the tip of your left index finger with the tip of your left index finger. That is why there is always an element of profound mystery in who we are.

We speak of confronting reality, facing the facts coming into this world. From birth we are trained to regard ourselves as being bags of skin facing outsiders in a world that is profoundly alien to us; we have a learned belief that what is outside of me is not me. This naturally sets up a fundamental sensation of hostility and estrangement between ourselves and the so-called external world, and leads us to talk of the conquest of nature, the conquest of space, and to view ourselves in a sort of battle stance with the world outside us.

Now all this is perfectly idiotic. A tree in the garden produces apples every summer and we call it an apple tree because the tree "apples"—that is what it does. Now, here is a solar system within a galaxy, and one of the peculiarities of this solar system is that, at least on the planet Earth, the thing "peoples" in just the same way as the apple tree apples. We grow out of this world in exactly the same way that the apples grow out of the apple tree. If evolution means anything, it means that.

WE AS ORGANISMS

The feeling that the external world is in some way a creation of the mind is very much in fashion today. It is a revival in Western philosophy of what used to be called *idealism*, a word referring to the metaphysical rather than the moral sense. But we come to this point of view with very different assumptions than those held by people like Hegel or Bishop Berkeley or Bradley, the great idealists of the European tradition.

The new idealism has a curiously physical basis. One is apt to hear that "everything you know is in your mind"; and that the distance, the feeling of externality, between you and other objects and people is also a content of consciousness; that therefore it is all your consciousness.

This has, of course, created all sorts of weird responses:

Are things there when I am not witnessing them,
or is anybody else there,
or are you all my personal dream?

One has only to imagine a conference of solipsists (those who believe that they alone exist) arguing as to which one of them is really there, to make the whole thing laughable! Furthermore, there seems to be no clarity in this kind of philosophical thinking as to what the terms *mind* or *consciousness* mean. Mind, soul and spirit have always been vague and formless images. Matter, by contrast, was very rugged, craggy. How these two influence each other no one could ever decide. All properly believed ghosts walk straight through brick walls without disturbing either the bricks or the ghost, so it has always been a mystery how a mind incarnate could move a material body.

In time people began to think that the differentiation between mind and matter was of no use. What happens when you make such a differentiation is that you impoverish both sides of it.

When you try to think of mind as immaterial, or matter as mindless, you get a king of mess on both sides.

It is the same with a mystic who is not a bit of a sensualist, or a sensualist who is not a bit of a mystic. Such a sensualist is boring, such a mystic is a fanatic, too spiritual.

It is the same when we divide the medical profession from the priesthood. Both are losers. This is not only because they have lost their opposite half. The problem is also that when you separate a doctor from a priest you do more than create two specializations out of what was originally one field. A priest-physician is more than a priest plus a physician. Having, as it were, binocular vision from medicine and from religion, the priest-physician sees not two areas, but one unified area in three dimensions.

In a similar way, when we have the concepts of mind

and matter working separately, both are impoverished. Mind becomes vague—kind of a psychic gas—and matter becomes mere stuff. Two sciences, biology and neurology, have enabled us to make a transition. Through biology, and to some extent physics, we have gotten the idea that man can be an objective observer of an external world that is not himself; that he can stand back from it and look at it and say what is out there.

Well, this cannot be done.

We can approximately do it, but we cannot really and fully do it, for two reasons.

The more important reason is that biologists show us very clearly that there is no way of definitively separating a human organism from its external environment. The two are a single field of behavior. Furthermore, to observe something alters it. This happens if you merely look at it, and the more so if you make experiments, "do science" on it. You cannot carry out observations without in some way interfering with what you observe. This is why we try to hide when, for instance, we are observing the habits and behavior of birds. When you watch something, it must not know you are looking.

Of course, what you ultimately want to do is to be able to watch yourself without knowing that you are looking! We want to catch ourselves not on our best behavior, and see ourselves as we really are. But this can never be done. Likewise, the physicist cannot simultaneously establish the position and velocity of very minute particles or "wavicles" because the experiment of observing nuclear behavior alters and affects what you are looking at.

The inseparability of human beings and their world deflates the myth of the objective observer standing aside and observing a world that is merely mechanical, operating like a machine *out there*.

The second reason that we cannot separate ourselves from the world around us grows out of the science of neurology. We understand clearly now that the kind of world we see is relative to the structure of the sense organ we use to perceive it. In other words, the qualities of the external world—its weight, color, texture, and so on—are possessed by it only in relation to a perceiving organism. The very structure of our optical system confers light and color upon outside energy.

We now have a new basis entirely for answering the old riddle: If a tree falls in the forest where no one is listening, does it make a noise? The answer in terms of modern science is perfectly clear. The falling tree creates vibrations in the air and these become noise if and only if they relate to an eardrum and an auditory nervous system.

In the same way, an ordinary drum, however hard you hit it, will make no sound if it has no skin. Sound is not something that exists in the external world. Sound is a relationship between vibrating air and certain kinds of biological organisms. It is these organisms that confer what we call sound upon a vibration, which in an earless world would make no noise. That is perfectly clear and straightforward. We can take certain steps from that.

Could we say, for example, that before any organisms existed there was no world?

When we posit a world prior to the existence of

organisms we are extrapolating. Let us talk about extrapolation for a moment.

Suppose you have a map of Kansas and you want, from the evidence contained in the map, to guess at what kind of territory lies beyond its edges. Naturally you will extend those straight-lined roads off and off and off. That is the only basis from which you can proceed. Nothing on the map of Kansas would warn you that a little way west you would encounter the Rocky Mountains, where the roads will have to wiggle. Still less would you have any warning that you are going to encounter the Pacific Ocean further on, which will not support any roads at all.

An extrapolation, then, is going from what is known to what is not known.

One might well wonder as to whether the existence of the universe before there were any living organisms is an extrapolation. We say this is how things would have been had we been around.

But we were not around.

Perhaps *it* was not around either.

This is a possible argument, but in today's climate of opinion it is not fashionable.

Watch out for fashion in philosophy, fashion in science. There are completely irrational functions that govern what is and what is not a respectable scientific opinion. Although very careful work is done and very valuable and thoughtful experimentation is carried out, in the background of this work there are always these irrational fashions of what is believable and what is not.

Many things that we accept today *were* completely unbelievable. We are always coming across this. There have been authoritative pronouncements that no one would ever reach the moon because of incontrovertible evidence of one kind or another.

But nowadays we have swung over to being a bit too uncritical. As Norbert Weiner warned in his book *Human Use of Human Beings*, we must not take science as a sort of fairy godmother and say, "Well, we have these problems of overpopulation and lack of water and so on, but science will solve it, don't worry." That is the other extreme.

The moment we accept metaphysical idealism we are saying that the way the world is is evoked by the structure of my own organism. In this way of thinking, all mountains and suns and moons and stars are the inhabitants of a strictly human world.

Perhaps insects, with their different sense organs, have a very different universe, an insect universe. This seems to be another manifestation of what used to be called the pathetic fallacy: the attribution of human qualities and emotions to natural phenomena.

The wind sighs in the trees and your heart is sad.

Then somebody comes along and says it is not the wind that is sighing, it is you.

True and not true.

You would not be able to sigh if there were no wind; you sighing and the wind blowing go together.

I have invented the new words *gowith* and *goeswith* to replace the idea of causality. Certain things gowith each other. Sighing wind goeswith the same world in which there are human hearts and emotions. If there were not a world with human hearts and emotions there would be no wind, and if there were no wind (air) there would be no human hearts and emotions; it is a transaction, a reciprocity.

In the same way, every event in the external world is dependent on the observer for its happening. Think of a rainbow. You can say that the sun is shining, there is moisture in the atmosphere, and the sun, being at the correct angle to the moisture, makes a rainbow. If the people are there, they see a rainbow. That is a way of putting things that is acceptable to us, in the current climate of philosophical and scientific fashion.

But I want to put it another way. The sun is shining and there is moisture in the air but there is no person present, so there is no rainbow. You must have all of the three elements—sun, moisture, and observer—to have the thing called rainbow. What applies to the tenuous, filmy, luminescent rainbow applies equally well to the hardest rocks, the most solid mountains, and the hottest fires.

All existence is a relationship.

Remember the importance of the skin of the drum. If it is not there, no amount of hitting the missing skin will produce any noise. We can see that energy is relationship: When we see the falling fish on the skin of the drum we know that if either were absent there would be no noise, no existence. We know that existence, however, is not only the impact of fist on drum.

Existence also requires a relationship with the neurological complex. Of course the neurological complex belongs to the same world as the sun. It is a physical pattern, physical behavior, physical energy. It takes this complexity of pattern to evoke the world.

This is a very simple idea to understand. The only difficulty is that it is unfamiliar and unfashionable.

As the rainbow metaphor illustrated, I arbitrarily favor an explanation of existence that is triadic. The impact of energies in the external world require an observer of this impact to energize or realize them (make them real).

You see, if the two forces out there are real and the observer is irrelevant to the reality of the situation, we are suddenly stuck with the notion that humankind itself is irrelevant. It is a notion that has had numerous supporters; humanity has always been conceived as irrelevant in various ways. Some may think us irrelevant because we are spiritual visitors from another world entirely. Others may consider us irrelevant because we are so small when measured against the size of the whole universe.

Now why do people want to think that humanity is irrelevant? What can people possibly achieve by taking this viewpoint?

It was fashionable in the nineteenth century to look upon human beings as irrelevant, for some very sound political reasons. When you are on the rampage you have to believe either that you are the representative of God Almighty and doing everything at His bidding or that what you are doing is not really very important. Either position will give you an alibi for behaving like a barbarian!

So the great put-down was invented, that our little affairs are of no concern to God ("Thank heaven, He's not watching anymore") and we can get away with murder. Which is what we wanted to do in the colonizations of the nineteenth century and the outrages of two world wars. There is no God watching anymore. God is dead, let's have a drink.

For a while Western man has lost his *place*—what the Hebrews used to call his position as the head of nature. People today will contend that man as the head of nature is the most conceited point of view; man is a part of nature, they say. But why is it that the naturalists, who think that man is a part of nature, are always fighting nature? It is because they do not understand what it means to be the head of nature.

Every creature, in its turn, is the head of nature. We all take turns, because it is taking turns that makes the world go around. Every creature is the head of nature because each creates the world in its own image. And so each creature as a creator of the world is man.

Man simply means the middle position; that is the whole idea of man. The middle, the middle way, the mean. And so, wherever the central point is, that is the point called man. Just as you are the center of your universe.

As the astrologists explain, to draw the map of a soul you take the center point occupied by the individual organism (in other words, the date and time of birth) to give you a latitude and a longitude. And on that date and time, how the universe was arranged shows the map of an individual soul. The individual is the whole universe considered from this point of view, or focused at this point of view.

In a like manner, the cosmic situation of a mouse

puts that mouse in the position of man when the mouse is considered the center of the universe.

Every point in a curved space-time continuum is the center of the universe. Although this is an imperfect metaphor, consider the surface of a sphere. Any point on that surface can be the center; just rotate it to what appears to be the "front" as you look at it, and that focal point becomes the center of the surface of the sphere.

It can be any point.

If our space is curved like the surface of the sphere, then any point on it may legitimately be considered the center.

That center point is called man.

As I say, it could be mouse, it could be ant, insect, anything.

But this becomes inconceivable and unimaginable to individuals who have no experience of themselves as center.

People who insist on the idea of being an objective observer—of watching the world as a kind of TV screen or movie upon which passes a distant panorama of events—by adopting that position exclude themselves from the feeling of centrality; in fact, they may well look down on the feeling of centrality. It has been called egotistic to think you are the center of everything. You may call it all sorts of bad names, you may call it the egocentric predicament, but that is the way it is. It is much less egocentric to accept it than to say, well, I'll go off and play my own game as an objective observer who is a sort of controller outside the world (in that qualitative sense in which the monotheistic God is said to be outside the world).

If you take this to its greatest extent, see how far you can go with it, then in the measure that you are the behavior of the universe, the universe is the behavior of you.

Earlier I mentioned the ease of understanding one way of looking at this, and the difficulty of understanding the other, even though one implies the other. When we see the degree to which individual behavior is a factor of the whole environmental scene, we tend to think that the individual organism is helplessly pushed around by, and responsive to, environmental forces.

On the other hand, if the relationship between the organism and its environment is *transactional*, it will not be one-sided. If the relationship is transactional, it will be true that simultaneously the individual organism behaves in accordance with the environment, and the environment behaves in accordance with the individual organism. To put that in startling practical terms:

If you go into a mess, that is what you wanted!

You may say, "I didn't know I wanted it, I didn't think I wanted it." This will be true, so long as you refer to yourself only in terms of the conscious spotlight which can experience bit by bit and actually thinks about it. But as soon as you extend your way of looking at things to include the unconscious, you find there may be underlying motivations not at first apparent.

This was clumsily foreshadowed by Freud and Jung, especially Freud with his ideas of self-punitiveness, death wishes, and so on. He held that when you get into a cat-astrophe it is because unconsciously you want to punish yourself. But Freud basically did not trust the uncon-scious. That is why he felt that the reality principle was in irreconcilable conflict with the pleasure principle and that this conflict would destroy human civilization.

Actually, a man named Georg Groddeck is much better at this than Freud; in *The Book of the It* he explains a most extraordinary theory of the unconscious. Throughout the whole thing he has complete faith in the unconscious and its wisdom. The book is in the form of letters from a goblin to a young girl. A friend to whom I lent it years ago said after reading it, "I will never be afraid of getting sick again," because Groddeck pointed out that sickness is not really a disease but a symptom of it, the unconscious, trying to cure you. Therefore, just as one does not simply knock down a fever with quinine because that would stop the work of the fever, so perhaps one should not knock down all sorts of diseases, if, for purposes which we do not yet under-stand, the unconscious is using them constructively.

This was something Freud was fumbling after: the notion that there is an intelligence in us greater than the intelligence of consciousness and operating in an uncon-scious way.

Note his choice of words. Why did Freud not say "superconscious"? Because the climate of opinion at the time he was alive wanted to insist that everything "below" human conscious reason was stupid, that mere matter, blind energy, had displaced God upon the throne of heaven. But Freud knew that you cannot eliminate the unconscious as part of your essential operation, your self.

Because you are an inseparable part of the world, you cannot "divvy up" responsibility and say, "You should praise me for that," "I should blame you for that," "It's your fault," and so on. Theologians are always talking a lot of nonsense about this kind of thing, saying that the dignity of man depends on each individual assuming his responsibility. And right away there is the free-for-all about who is to blame for everything.

Now, if you understand that you are an integral functioning part of this whole cosmos, the price you have to pay to stop all this nattering about blame is to admit your own complicity in the catastrophes that have occurred to you. You must see that everything that comes to you is a return of everything that went out of you.

You asked for it.

But it is not the *conscious* you that asked for it. Not the you that is just spotlight consciousness, because that is unaware of most of the things that go on in you. There are curious and fascinating things operating underneath the surface of your consciousness.

There is much to be gained from studying some science. Take an elementary course in ecology for example. You will see a developing pattern in which everything from microscopic organisms onward gets integrated into the whole thing that is going on. What from one point of view is the disease of a certain plant is the method of reproduction of some other species. We say that we get malaria from anopheles mosquitoes, but it is because the anopheles mosquito has an extraordinary reproductive cycle that involves its being parasitic to humans. If you were to take the anopheles' point of view, it becomes man.

As we study the various systems we find that everything is in a constant state of adjustment. If you were to examine the edge of a leaf under a microscope you would find a constant churning, churning going on. Some of the cells want to move way out there, and if they do the leaf starts to disintegrate. But some other cells come along and say, "Get back inside, keep in, keep in," and the original ones say, "No, you are destroying our liberty, we want to get out," and this whole clamor goes on at the edge of a leaf. But from our point of view it is a perfectly stable, clean edge; we are not looking closely enough.

I once saw a great plant covered with greenflies; they were succulent and fat and having a ball. I came by the next day and the whole thing was gray dust. They had eaten up the plant and disintegrated. As a fact of nature, we say thank heavens for those greenflies; they just ate up the weed and both of them were pests anyway. They represent the balancing system of nature.

We are, doubtless, in the same situation, only we have some kind of blinkers on whereby we only see half the picture.

We get the idea that "it" can push us around, but we do not get the idea that being pushed around is what we asked for. We evoked it by the very fact that we are here.

Children do not think they are responsible for being born. They blame their parents, not realizing that they cannot really separate themselves from their parents. For example, in the measure that I have sexual desires I can really understand my father's predicament, and I could not possibly blame him, because actually I was the gleam in his eye when he approached my mother. You know, I asked for it!

Now, you can see in this that your relationship to the world, being responsible for everything that happens to you, is not that of an ordinary boss who might decree that all sorts of improbable things should happen.

Rather it is this.

If you think of yourself only as the consciousness and being in control of everything that happens to you, you will act stupidly, like a kind of lunatic thinking he is God. If, on the other hand, you understand that your real self is the wisdom that is expressed in the intelligent form of your organism, you will not fall into the error of thinking your relationship to the world is that of being its governor.

Who Am I?

Really, the fundamental, ultimate mystery, the only thing you need to know to understand the deepest metaphysical secrets is this: For every outside there is an inside, and for every inside there is an outside, and although they are different, they go together. There is, in other words, a secret conspiracy between all insides and all outsides, and the conspiracy is this: To look as different as possible and yet underneath to be identical, because you do not find one without the other.

I and my environment and you and your environment are explicitly as different as different can be, but implicitly we go together. And this is discovered by the scientist when he tries to describe what happens exactly, which is the art of science. When he describes exactly what you do, he finds out that you, your behavior, is not something that can be separated from the behavior of the world around you. He realizes then that you are something that the whole world is doing. Just as when the sea has waves on it—the sea, the ocean, is "waving"—so each one of us is a "waving" of the whole cosmos.

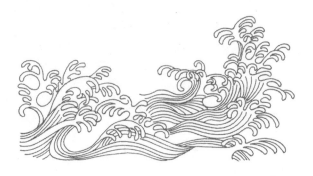

OM CREATIVE MEDITATIONS

INTELLECTUAL YOGA

The word *yoga*, as you may know, is the same as the English word *yoke* and the Latin word *jungare* (to join). When Jesus said, "My yoke is easy," he was also saying, "My *yoga* is easy." Yoga describes the state that is the opposite of what our psychologists call alienation, the feeling of separateness, of being cut off from being.

Many civilized people do in fact feel alienated, because they have a kind of myopic attention focused on their own boundaries and what is inside those boundaries. They identify themselves with the inside, not realizing that you cannot have an inside without an outside.

That would seem to be extremely elementary logic. We could have no sense of being ourselves, of having a personal identity, without the contrast of something that is not ourselves, is *other*.

Not realizing that *self* and *other* go together is the root of an enormous and terrifying anxiety caused by wondering what will happen when the inside disappears.

What will happen when the so-called *I* comes to an end, as it seems to?

Of course, if things did not keep moving and changing, appearing and dissolving, the universe would be a colossal bore. Therefore you are only aware that things are all right for the moment.

You must realize that the sense of life's being fairly all right is inconceivable and unfeelable unless there is—way, way back in your mind—the glimmer of a possibility that something absolutely, unspeakably awful might happen. It does not *have* to happen, because you may die first, but there always has to be the vague apprehension that the awful awfuls are possible. It gives spice to life.

These observations relate to the intellectual approach to yoga.

There are certain principal forms of yoga with which most people are familiar. Hatha-yoga is a psychophysical exercise system; it is the one you see demonstrated on TV because it has visual value.

Then there is bhākti yoga; *bhākti* means devotion. I suppose you might say that Christianity is a form of bhākti-yoga, because it is yoga practiced through extreme reverence for and love for some being felt more or less external to oneself who is the representative of the divine.

Then there is karma-yoga. *Karma* means action—and incidentally, that is all it means. It does not mean the law of cause and effect.

When we say something that happens to you
   is your karma,
all it means is that it is your own doing.
Nobody is in charge of your karma except you.

Karma-yoga is the way of action, of using your everyday life, your trade, or an athletic discipline like sailing, surf riding, or running as your way of yoga, your way of discovering who you are.

Rāja-yoga, the royal yoga that is sometimes called kundalini-yoga, involves very complicated psychic exercises having to do with awakening the serpent power that is supposed to lie at the base of one's spiritual spine, raising it up through certain chakras (or centers) until it enters the brain. (There is a very profound symbolism involved in this but we won't go into it here.)

There are several other yogas, then finally there is mantra-yoga. Mantra-yoga is the practice through chanting or humming, either aloud or silently, certain sounds which become supports for contemplation, or what in Sanskrit is called *dhyāna*.

Dhyāna is the state in which one is clearly awake and aware of the world as it is, as distinct from the world as it is described. In other words, in the state of dhyāna you stop thinking. That is to say, you stop talking to yourself and symbolizing to yourself what is going on.

You simply are aware of what is.

And nobody can say what it is, because as someone once said, "The real world is unspeakable."

Sitting absolutely wide awake with eyes open but not thinking is a very curious state, incidentally. I knew a professor of mathematics at Northwestern University who once said, "You know it is amazing how many things there are that aren't so." He was talking about old wives' tales and superstitions and so on. But when you practice dhyāna you are amazed at how many things are not so.

When you stop talking to yourself and are simply

aware of what is, that is to say, of what you feel, what you sense (even that is saying too much), you suddenly find that the past and the future have completely disappeared.

Also, the so-called differentiation between the knower and the known, the subject and the object, the feeler and the feeling, the thinker and the thought has disappeared. They are not there because you have to talk to yourself to maintain those things. They are purely conceptual; they are ideas, phantoms, ghosts.

When you allow thinking to stop, all that goes away, and you find that you are in an eternal here and now. There is nowhere you are supposed to be, nothing you are supposed to do, nowhere you are supposed to go, because in order to think you must do something, you have to *think*.

It is incredibly important to *unthink* at least once a day, for the very preservation of intellectual life. If you do nothing but think, as you are advised by most of the academic teachers and gurus, you will have nothing to think about except thoughts. You can easily become like a great university library, which is very often a place where people bury themselves to write books about the books that are already there. They write books about books about books and the library swells like an enormous batch of yeast, and that is all that is going on.

It is a very amusing game. I love to bury my nose in ancient Oriental texts, for instance. It is fun; it is like playing poker or chess, or doing pure mathematics. But the trouble is that it gets increasingly unrelated to life because the thinking is all words about words.

If we stop that temporarily and get our minds clear

of thoughts, we "become again as children" and get a direct view of the world which is very useful when you are an adult.

There is not much you can do when you are a baby because everybody pushes you around. They pick you up and put you down, and you cannot do much except practice contemplation! You cannot tell anyone what it is like.

But when, as an adult, you can recapture the baby's point of view, you will know what all child psychologists have always wanted to know:

How a baby feels.

The baby, according to Freud at least, has *oceanic* experience; that is to say, a feeling of complete inseparability from what is going on. The baby is unable to distinguish between the universe and its own action upon the universe.

And most of us, if we got into that state of consciousness, might be inclined to feel extremely frightened and begin to ask who is in charge. Who controls what happens next? We would ask that because we are used to the idea that the process of nature consists of controllers and controllees—things that do and things that are done to. This is purely mythological, as you find out when you observe the world without thinking, with a purely silent mind.

There is an intellectual way to get at this kind of understanding; jnāna-yoga is the approach to that which is intellectual. People often say to me, "I understand what you are talking about intellectually, but I don't really feel it, I don't realize it," and I am apt to reply, "I wonder whether you do understand it intellectually, because if you did you would also feel it."

The intellect, what I prefer to call the intelligence, is not a sort of watertight compartment of the mind that goes clickety-clickety all by itself and has no influence on what happens in all other spheres of one's being. We all know you can be hypnotized by words. Certain words immediately arouse certain feelings. By using certain words it is very easy to change people's emotions. They are incantations.

The intellect is not something separate out there. But the word *intellect* has become a kind of clickety, a word that represents the intellectual "porcupinism" of the academic world. As a certain professor said at Harvard at the time Tim Leary was doing experiments there, "No knowledge is academically respectable that cannot be put into words." (Alas for the department of physical education; alas for the departments of music and fine arts!)

One of the greatest intellectuals of modern time, Ludwig Wittgenstein, at the end of his greatest book *Tractatus*, shows you that what you always thought were major problems in life and philosophy were meaningless questions. And that those problems are solved not by giving an answer to them, but by getting rid of the problem through seeing intellectually that it is meaningless. Then you are *relieved* of the problem. You need no longer lie awake nights wondering what is the meaning of life, what it is all about. Simply because it is not about anything. It is about itself.

And so Wittgenstein ends by saying, "Whereof one cannot speak, thereof one must be silent."

There are certain things of which one cannot speak.

For example, you cannot *describe* music. That is why most of the reports of music critics in the newspaper seem completely absurd. When they are trying to convey in words how a certain artist performs, they borrow words from all other kinds of art and try to make some show of being clever about it. But there is no way in which the music critic can, through words, make you hear the sounds of the concert.

However, by writing certain instructions on paper, telling you certain things to do, these sounds can be reproduced. Musical notation is essentially a set of instructions (just like "scribe a circle" or "drop a perpendicular"). And so, if you follow the instructions, then you will understand the things that cannot be described. That is what yoga is all about.

All mystical writing really is instructions. It is not an attempt to describe the universe, to describe God, to describe ultimate reality. Every mystic knows that cannot possibly be done. The very word *mysticism* is from the Greek word *myein* which means keeping silence.

Be quiet, see, then you will understand, because the instructions are to listen, to look. Stop, look, and listen—and see what is going on—that is yoga. Only don't say,

don't say...

that will spoil it.

Somebody came to a Zen master and said, "The

mountains and the hills and the sky, are not all these the body of Buddha?"

And the master said, "Yes, but it is a pity to say so."

A new successor to Wittgenstein, an Englishman named Spencer Brown, has written a book called *Law of Form* which allows those who are mathematically oriented to go through an intellectual process that is very close indeed to jnāna-yoga. Brown begins with the instruction to the reader to draw a distinction, any distinction you want, between something and nothing, between the inside and the outside, what have you. Then he leads you through a process of reasoning where he shows you that, once you have made that step, all the laws of mathematics, physics, biology, and electronics follow inexorably. He draws them all out. He gets you into immensely complicated electronic circuitry systems that necessarily follow from your having drawn a distinction. Once you have done that, the universe as we know it is inevitable. Afterwards he says that he has not told you anything you did not know already. At every step, when you saw that one of his proofs (his theorems) was correct, you said, "Oh, of course," because you knew it already.

Then at the end of it, where he has shown you, as it were, the nature of your own mind, he raises the question, "Was this trip really necessary?"

So now he takes us on a reentry and says, "You see what has happened through all this mathematical process, and also in the course of your complicated lives, where you have been trying to find something: The universe has taken one turn."

That is the meaning of the uni-verse. It has taken a turn on itself. To look at itself.

Now, when anything looks at itself it escapes itself. Like the snake swallowing its tail or the dog chasing its tail, it gets some of it, but does not get *it*.

And so Brown makes the amazing remark, "Naturally as our telescopes become more powerful, the universe must expand in order to escape them."

Now, you will say that this is subjective idealism in a new disguise, this is Bishop Berkeley all over again, saying that we created the universe out of our own minds. Well, unfortunately this is true. If you take mind to mean brain, physical brain, physical nervous system, you will find Karl Pribram of Stanford saying the same thing in neurological terms. It is the structure of your nervous system which causes you to see the world that you see. You may prefer to read J. Z. Young's book *Doubt and Certainty in Science* where all of this is very clearly explained in newer, more scientifically respectable language. But it is the same old thing.

That is yoga, you see. Yoga, union, means that

you do it.

In a sense, you are God. You are making it.

Many spiritual teachers and gurus will look at their disciples and say, "I am God, I have realized. See?" But the important thing is that *you* are.

Whether I am God is of no consequence to you whatsoever. I could tell you, "I have realized," or put on a turban and a yellow robe and approach you saying, "I am guru, you need the grace of guru in order to realize," and it would be a wonderful hoax. It would be like picking your pockets and selling you your own watch!

The point is, you are.

Now, what are we saying when we say that? Obviously something very important.

Alas, there is no way of defining it, going any further into words about it. When a philosopher hears such a statement as "you are it" or "there is only the eternal now" he is inclined to say, "Well, I don't see why you are so excited about it. What do you mean by that?" He asks the question because he wants to continue the word game and he does not want to go on into an experiential dimension. He wants to go on arguing because that is his trip.

Words have meaning because they are symbols, because they point to something other than themselves. But all of these great mystical statements mean nothing whatsoever because they are ultimate, just as the clouds and the mountains and the stars have no *meaning* because they are not *words*. The stars and the clouds are like music. Only bad music has any meaning; classical music never has a meaning. To understand it you simply listen to it, observing its beautiful patterns and going into its complexities.

So when your mind—that is, your verbal systems— get to the end of their tether, when they arrive at the meaningless statement, that is the critical point. The method of jnāna-yoga is to exercise your intellect to its limits until you reach the point where you have no fur- ther questions to ask.

You can do this in the study of philosophy if you

have the right kind of teacher, who shows you that all philosophical opinions whatsoever are false—or at the least, extremely partial. You can see how the nominalists cancel out the realists. How the determinists cancel out the free-willists. How the behaviorists cancel out the vitalists. How the logical positivists cancel out everybody! And then somebody comes along and asserts that the logical positivists have concealed metaphysics, which indeed they do. And then you get into an awful tangle and there is nothing for you to believe.

If you get seriously into the study of theology and comparative religion, exactly the same thing can happen to you. You cannot be an atheist anymore. That is also shown to be a purely mythological position, and so you feel a kind of intellectual vertigo which is called in a Zen Buddhist poem:

> "Above not a tile to cover the head,
> below not an inch of ground to stand on."

Where are you then? Well, of course, you are where you always were.

You have discovered you are IT.

And that is very uncomfortable because you cannot grab IT.

You have discovered that whatever it is that you are (and it is not something inside your head, it is as much out there as it is in here), you cannot get ahold of it. Well, that gives you the heebie-jeebies, you get butterflies in your stomach, anxiety traumas, and all kinds of things.

But this is all explained by Shankara, the great

Hindu commentator upon the Upanishads, the great master of the nondualistic doctrine of the universe, when he says, "That which knows, which is in all beings the knower, is never the object of its own knowledge."

To everyone who is in quest of the supreme kick, the great experience, the vision of God, liberation—whatever you want to call it—when you think that you are not IT, any old guru can sell you on a method to find it. And that may not be a bad thing for the guru to do, because as Blake said, "A fool who persists in his folly will become wise." And a clever guru is a person who leads you on.

"Here, kitty, kitty, kitty...I've got something very good to sell you, you just wait; but you have to go through a lot of stages yet."

And you say, "(pant, pant, pant) Can I get that? Oh, I want to get that!" And all the time IT is you.

I was talking to a Zen master the other day and he said, "You shall be my disciple."

I looked at him and said, "Who was Buddha's teacher?"

He looked at me in a very odd way for a moment and then he burst into laughter and handed me a piece of clover.

So you see, as long as you can be persuaded that there is something more you ought to be than you are, you have divided yourself from reality, from the universe, from God, whatever you want to call it.

And you will find repeatedly, if you are interested in these things, that in psychoanalysis, in gestalt therapy, in sensitivity training, in any kind of yoga, or what have you, there will be this peculiar sensation of spiritual greed that can be aroused by somebody indicating to you, "Hmmm, there are still higher stages for you to attain. You should meet my guru."

You might say that to be truly realized you have to get to the point where you are not seeking anymore. So then you begin to think, "Well, I will now be a non-seeker."

This amounts to becoming spiritually unspiritual. You will find that is what is called in Zen "legs on a snake." It is irrelevant. You don't need not to seek. You don't need anything.

A Buddhist scholar named Nogaguna, who lived about A.D. 200, invented a whole dialectic and found a school where the "leader" of the students would simply destroy all of their ideas—absolutely abolish their philosophic notions. And they would get the heebie-jeebies and see that the leader did not have the heebie-jeebies, that he seemed perfectly relaxed in having no particular point of view. "Teacher how can you stand it? We have to have something to hold on to." And the teacher's response: "Who does? Who are you?"

Eventually, of course, they discovered that it is not necessary to hang onto anything, to rely on anything. There is nothing to rely on because you are IT. It is like asking the question "Where is the universe?"

Where is it in space? Everything in it is falling around everything else, but there is no concrete floor underneath for the thing to crash upon, because space goes out and out forever and ever and has no end.

What is that? What else could it be?

Of course, it is you.

Only the universe is delightfully arranged so that it looks at itself, in order not to be one-sided and prejudiced, from innumerable points of view.

Now, if you understand what I am saying with your intelligence, but you do not feel it, I must ask why you want to feel it. You may say, "I want something more," but that again is spiritual greed, and you only say that because you did not understand it.

There is nothing to pursue because you are IT. To put it in Christian or Jewish terms, if you do not know you are God from the beginning, what happens is that you try to become God by force. You start by being violent and obstreperous.

All our violence, all our competitiveness, all our terrific anxiety to survive is because we did not know from the beginning that we were IT.

If we had known from the beginning, some people will say, then nothing would ever have happened.

But it did happen, didn't it?

Let me tell you, if you do by chance find out who you really are, instead of becoming lazy, you start laughing, laughing leads to dancing, dancing leads to music, and we can play with each other for a change.

Who Am I?

People who, by various means, become fully aware of their universal consciousness have what is called a mystical experience or a cosmic consciousness. The Buddhists call it awakening. The Hindus call it liberation, because they discover that the real, deep self—that which you are fundamentally and forever—is the whole of being. All that there is, the works, that is you.

Only that universal self that is you has the capacity to focus itself on ever so many different here-and-nows. So when you use the word "I," it is, as William James said, really a word of position, like "this" or "here." Just as a sun or star has many rays, so the whole cosmos expresses itself in each of us with all our different variations. The cosmos dances with infinite variety. But every single dance it does, that is to say "you," is what the whole thing is doing.

LANDSCAPE, SOUNDSCAPE, AND THE WATERCOURSE WAY

For thousands of years the arts of painting and sculpture served mainly religious purposes. There was really no such thing as what we now call fine art. All art was iconographic and functional, intended to be used for contemplation, ritual, or magic. In a museum devoted to ancient art (or, indeed, to any art pre-Renaissance) almost every exhibit will be something of religious or magical function. The art will consist principally of effigies of human or divine animal figures.

In painting, of course, you cannot see a figure without a background. (As a matter of fact, that is also true of sculpture, but in our culture we have considered the background in sculpture irrelevant because it is not something which the artist created.) But when you paint, especially when you paint on a rectangular surface instead of one shaped so that the outline of the figure is also the frame, you must put in some kind of background.

Early Greek or Russian icons had backgrounds of solid gold, often emblazoned with jewels. But as time went on, painters began to put landscape in the backgrounds of their paintings, because that is the way we see people. They must be seen *against* something.

In due course, Western painters began to be fascinated with the background. In effect they said to the figure, "Move over," and landscape painting was born. People seeing these landscapes who were not used to the idea said, "Well, that's not my idea of a painting."

But in time they got used to it. Now, in fact, people are so used to landscape that in every national park you will find a place called Inspiration Point. Tourists come from far away to gaze at it and say, "Oh, it is just like a picture."

A very mysterious thing has happened. What was it that came to intrigue painters about mountains, trees, clouds, and rivers? Why did they begin to see them as beautiful? Why, suddenly, did they get this vision that these things were worth copying?

All of a sudden painters were falling in love with the nonsymmetrical. Human and animal forms, although wiggly, are more or less symmetrical. We look as if we had been folded down the middle; we have an eye on either side, two ears, two arms, two legs, and we do look pretty symmetrical. But clouds don't. The nonsymmetrical has an air of freedom about it.

Then there is another thing. We worry about our behavior a great deal. We talk about good behavior and bad behavior, sane behavior and crazy behavior, artificial behavior and natural behavior; we have a big thing about this.

But the painter does not worry about the behavior of clouds or of spraying water or rocks. It would be unimaginable to accuse a wave of making an aesthetic mistake. Nobody has ever, I think, drawn an objection to a badly formed cloud. And only once in history was there a complaint about the stars. There was a Frenchman in the eighteenth century who criticized the Lord for not arranging the stars in fine geometrical patterns that would be edifying to the intellect, but instead scattering them at random across the sky! That was during the period when people were making formal gardens, clipping trees and hedges into the shapes of birds and animals, and laying out the plantings and walks in precise geometrical forms.

If you were to fly across the United States from San Francisco to New York, you would first encounter a long stretch of mountain country where human beings must, perforce, accord with nature.

By and large, all the roads are curly because they have to go along mountain valleys. There are curly rivers and wonderful washes, which, interestingly, are in the form of trees. (It is really fascinating that rivers and trees are the same shape. The flow of sap in the tree and the flow of water in the river are both analogous to the flow of life.)

There is a watercourse character to the formations you see as you fly eastward. They all wiggle, just as the roads wiggle until you get to Denver. After Denver, where the country is flat, everything goes straight. It is laid out in rectangles, Euclidean, squared away by humans. The land reflects our passion, even compulsion, to straighten things out.

We say, "Let's get things straightened out."

Why?

Would it not be more fun to make things more curvaceous, rather than to straighten them out?

For example, the fundamental movement of dancing is where the hips move independently of the shoulders. When you watch Hindu dancers, their arms are going in that rhythm of the hips and shoulders and they look as if they were in water. They look like water plants moving in the current, and many of us think that is very beautiful. Really wiggly human behavior.

It brings us back to the water. There is a watercourse character to all the forms that emerge in space.

If you study water flow, you get what is really basic to nature. Lao-tse, writing a little before 500 B.C., pointed out that the course of nature, the *tao*, is like water. Extremely soft, water overcomes all hard things; in being weak it is strong; it always seeks the lowest level, the path of least resistance.

Western people have been taught that to go with nature, to take the path of least resistance, is unmanly, spineless, weak-kneed, and altogether wrong. We are all brought up to be energetic and aggressive, to use force. A child who is not forceful in school is likely to be reported by the teachers as at least mildly defective. This is really wrongheaded.

In thinking about human affairs, always call common sense into question. It is the most creative part of philosophy. Take ideas which are commonly accepted and which seem to be incontrovertible and question them. Turn them inside out and see what would happen if they were thought about in another way.

For example, everyone automatically assumes that the present is the result of the past. Turn it around, and consider whether the past may not be a result of the present. The past may be streaming back from the now, like the country as seen from an airplane.

If you look at it that way it makes sense. Just as the tail does not wag the dog, the past does not cause the present—unless you insist that it does.

Actually, the whole universe emerges from the present. It is all beginning now. We are present at this moment at the beginning of creation, and the past is simply echoes going back through the corridors of our minds.

The past is, in fact, present.

You see, the universe is a vibration.

It seems to us still and solid, like a rock. We are not normally aware that the rock is an extremely fast vibration, so fast that we cannot see the intervals between the vibrations.

Actually, everything is going on and off; it is an electronic performance. The world is coming at us like a movie. It is all coming out of space. We see the stars vibrating out of space; if there were not space, there could not be stars or galaxies.

But now we see that something is coming out of nothing.

It is perfectly obvious that nothing is the root of something. You cannot have something without nothing. You cannot have the figure without the background.

The hollow and the solid come into being together.

Lao-tse says, "To be and not to be arise mutually." The yang and the yin principles create each other. They are likened to the northern and southern sides of a mountain: the north side, the shade; the south side, the sun. Obviously you cannot have a mountain with only one side.

Human beings who do not perceive this principle are always trying to have the yang without the yin. They want the light without the dark, the good without the bad, the pleasurable without the painful, the something without the nothing, the life without the death. This, of course, is profoundly illogical.

All of this yang/yinning has within it a *pattern,* and this pattern is revealed in the flow of water and how it behaves. Artists have sought to copy it because in water it is shown that the *tao,* or the course of nature, never makes an aesthetic mistake.

The fellow who complained to God that the stars were badly arranged lacked an adequate perspective of this galaxy. We are in the galaxy and close up it does look as if the stars are randomly scattered. But if we were to go away to a tremendous distance we could see that this galaxy is beautifully formed as a double helix. Many other galaxies are also magnificent double helixes, although they have varying shapes. In a double helix we find that the two elements are spiraling about, chasing after each other. And the one does not know itself except in terms of the other.

You would not be aware of the sensation of self unless at the same time you were aware of the sensation of something other. You cannot see figure without background.

Now, if you cannot have self without other, yang without yin, front without back, or the knowledge of voluntary action without the experience of what involuntarily happens, then there is a conspiracy going on. In other words, there are two which *appear* to be different, yet they are esoterically and secretly the same.

When you come to know that, you have a problem. This is why one could say that being enlightened in the Buddhist sense of the word is a sort of calamity. You find out the ruse you were playing on yourself. You find out that the universe is a system that creeps up on itself and says, "Boo!" and then laughs at itself for jumping.

The universe is a self-surprising arrangement, so as to avoid the monotony and boredom of knowing everything in advance. And you and I have conspired with ourselves to pretend that we are not really God.

But of course we are.

We are all apertures through which the universe is looking at itself.

Perhaps because artists were beginning to have a glimmer of this, at a certain point in the development of painting, they began to tire of copying people, trees, clouds, and water, and asked themselves why *they* could not create works of nature.

And so they did.

Jackson Pollock, in dripping paint on canvas, actually let this watercourse thing happen without copying anything. The artist must be in a certain state to do this, because there is something fundamentally different between fine abstract painting and mere mess.

A lot of people thought that any child could do abstract painting, so they set out to make abstract paintings that no one found interesting because they were just terrible. And some people took typewriters and hit them several times with a sledgehammer and then mounted them on blocks of walnut and called them "Opus 14" or whatever. And they were completely phony.

But it was obvious that Pollock and many other abstract artists were not phonies, though it was impossible to explain why.

In the same way it is impossible to explain why the patterns in water, clouds, or mountains are beautiful.

The instructor of a course in aesthetics might draw a series of triangles over a painting and call attention to the patterns which hold your eye, but that is mere geometry and it is absolute foolishness to contend that the beauty lies solely in the geometry. Nobody knows, or can possibly say, why a mountain is beautiful. In art schools where they try to teach one to do beautiful things, they eventually find that beauty is unteachable. If it were teachable, we would have thousands of Rembrandts and Picassos emerging from art schools and people would say, "Oh, this is old hat, let's have something new."

It is equally true that music cannot be taught. What you can teach is how to play an instrument, how to write notation. You can copy the old masters, but you are still just copying. When Bach wrote music, he really invented the laws of harmony. Now everybody studies Bach to find out what the laws of harmony are.

In the same way, language comes along before grammar. A child picks up language by ear, and on going to school is amazed and horrified to discover this language has grammar. Lots of people in the world did not know they had grammar until some anthropologist told them, having discovered the rules of their so-called primitive languages.

So the artist does not know what constitutes beauty for exactly the same reason that you and I cannot see our own heads and do not know how our brains work. Even the greatest neurologists do not know how the brain works and they are the first to admit it. They do not know how we manage to be conscious, how we make decisions; we just do it, in the same way we move our fingers without knowing any physiology. Also, in the same way, the artist manages to create the beautiful.

One may suppose, therefore, that someday when spontaneous painting has come to be understood by the masses, people will walk down city streets and stop before filthy walls covered with scraps of torn-off posters, bird droppings, and scratches to say, "Oh, it is just like a picture."

Let us take a look at Western music. Consider what a ritual a Western concert is. There are all these ladies and gentlemen wearing black clothes sitting in a great semi-circle; the conductor arrives to tremendous hullabaloo and bows and motions to the orchestra; suddenly he is ready to go. And then this *thing* begins. It may be 4/4 time or 6/8 time, but it will be a regular beat. Though it may be a sentimental and melodic piece, to the Oriental ear it will sound like a military march. And it is *very* serious. The musicians are doing the *thing* that we are supposed to listen to, and all other sounds are to be suppressed. You do not see the orchestra members laughing at each other as they do in, say, a Hindu orchestra. The audience must be silent, no coughing, blowing noses, shuffling feet, because there is this *thing* to listen to.

The same sort of thing goes on in radio and television studios, where they will go to incredible lengths to pretend that they are not on the radio or on TV. Surrounded by soundproof walls, someone counts down with a clock and says, "Stand by," and everybody has to be silent. Then he points to the main speaker and says, "Go." It would be a terrible faux pas to have extraneous sounds intrude during the program. But when you are listening to the radio or watching TV, you may also be hearing a crackling fire, a truck going by, or somebody typing. Why then all this concern about eliminating noise?

John Cage, an extremely competent musician and a good friend of mine, is an extraordinary eccentric. First he experimented with opening up the piano and attaching paperclips, nails, and washers to the strings so that they made very unusual noises.

Then he played regular set pieces with what he called his prepared-piano.

Then he decided he would set up a row of twelve radios, each with an operator, and according to a series of intervals derived from the *I Ching*, they would turn the radios on and off. As the radios were all set on different stations, the effect was of an extraordinary battle.

Next he tape-recorded all kinds of sounds: traffic, people, airports, and so on, and he played them all at once.

Another time he recorded an enormous amount of

miscellaneous noise and played it in an art gallery where people were milling around; he recorded the happening itself, the noise made by the audience in reaction to all the noise he had prepared originally. He played that back to them, re-recorded their reaction to it, and then played that back.

Then he thought of a really amazing idea. He gave a formal concert in one of the major halls in New York City. Cage appeared beautifully dressed in white tie and tails with an assistant to turn the pages of the score at the grand piano. Everything was very formally set up. But the score consisted entirely of rests. It had a key signature and repeat places which required turning the page back. Cage sat down at the piano and waited the proper time of the thing while the man turned the pages and the audience began to titter and shuffle and cough and sneeze. The point of the performance was for the audience to listen to itself. He did not explain this, but the word had got around that this was the idea.

You see, what he was doing was to draw attention to the *soundscape*. Just as landscape is the natural background of people, buildings and so on, so the background of music is soundscape, the susurrus of sound going on all over the place.

There is a certain importance to this, and we must go to Chinese philosophy to understand it.

The Chinese developed landscape long before we did. As early as A.D. 700, there were landscape painters in China. When human figures appeared in landscape they were very tiny, because the Chinese always saw humans in the context of nature. They did not see the organism except in relation to its environment. They also had a different concept of perspective. Our convention of perspective is that things become smaller as they are farther away from you (and presumably less important). Many people who are not part of our culture, when shown a perspective drawing, do not comprehend it at all. They point out that the tree there in the distance is not that small in relation to something in the foreground; they just do not see it as we do.

Once, when an American G.I. was visiting Picasso during the Liberation of France, he said that he could not understand the artist's paintings. "Why do you paint a person looking from the side and from the front at the same time?"

Picasso asked, "Do you have a girlfriend?"

"Yes," replied the soldier.

"Do you have a picture of her?" The soldier pulled from his wallet a photograph of the girl.

Picasso looked at it in mock astonishment and asked, "Is she so small?"

What we think about art and about life depends, to an enormous extent, on convention. But we must beware of phony spontaneity, of merely going against convention. That is not the watercourse way. That is not the line of least resistance.

We must be very sensitive to discover what that line is.

When we have done so,
then we are able to flow.

Who Am I?

When we feel that we understand something, most of us really mean that we have managed to translate it into words. However, we understand an enormous number of things that we do not know about in words. We understand how to breathe, for instance, but we are not able to put it into words.

Somehow we have gotten ourselves into the frame of mind where, unless we can put something into words—especially the kind of thing that I have been discussing—we feel that we do not understand it. There are whole ways of life that cannot be contained within the networks that we regard as sensible or academically respectable. This includes the ways of life of plants. We say of somebody whose body and mind scarcely function that they have become a mere vegetable. That is a very insulting thing to say about vegetables. No vegetable is a "mere" vegetable.

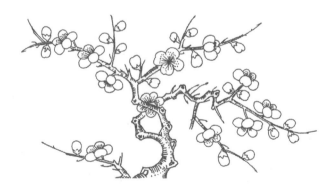

SHE IS BLACK

There is an old story about the astronaut who went far out into space and was asked upon his return whether he had been to heaven and seen God.

"Yes," he said.
"Well, what about God?"
"She is black."

Though this is a well-worn story, it is very profound.

I knew a monk who started out in life as an agnostic. Then he began to read Henry Bergson, the French philosopher who proclaimed the vital force (*élan vital*). The more he read into this kind of philosophy, the more he saw that these people were really talking about God.

I myself have read a great deal of theological reasoning about the existence of God, and it all starts out along this line: If you are intelligent and reasonable, you cannot be a product of a mechanical and meaningless universe. Figs do not grow on thistles, grapes do not grow on thorns; therefore you, as an expression of the universe, as an aperture through which the universe is observing itself, cannot be a mere fluke.

Because if this world *peoples*, as trees bring forth fruit, then the universe itself—the energy which underlies it, what it is all about—must be intelligent.

Now, when you come to that conclusion, you must be very careful, because you may make an unwarranted jump to the further conclusion that that intelligence, that marvelous designing power which produces all of this, is the Biblical God.

Be careful.

Because that God, contrary to His own commandments, is fashioned in the graven image of a paternal, authoritative, beneficent tyrant of the ancient Middle East. It is very easy to fall into that trap because it is all prepared, institutionalized in the Roman Catholic Church, in the synagogue, in the Protestant churches—all there ready for you to accept.

Under the pressure of social consensus it is very natural to assume that when somebody uses the word *God*, it is that father figure which is intended, because even Jesus used the analogy of the father for his experience of God.

He *had* to, there was no other one available to him in his culture.

Nowadays we are in rebellion against the image of the authoritarian father. This is especially true in the United States, which is a republic rather than a monarchy. But to reject the paternalistic image of God as an idol is not necessarily to be an atheist.

I have advocated something called atheism in the name of God. That is to say, an experience, a contact, a relationship to God with the ground of your being, that does not have to be embodied or expressed in any specific image. Theologians, on the whole, do not like that idea.

I find in my discourse with them that they want to be a little bit hard-nosed about the nature of God. They want to say that God has, indeed, a very specific nature. This ethical monotheism holds that the governing power of this universe has some extremely definite opinions and rules to which our minds and acts must be conformed. If you do not watch out, you will go against the fundamental grain of the universe and be punished. In old-fashioned parlance, you will burn in the fires of hell forever. In modern terms, you will fail to be an authentic person. (It is just another way of talking about it.)

There is this feeling that there is this *authority* behind the world and it is not you, it is something else. This approach, which is Judeo-Christian, and indeed Muslim, makes a lot of people feel estranged from the root and ground of being. There are, in fact, a lot of people who never grow up and who are always in awe of the image of grandfather.

Now I am a grandfather and I am no longer in awe of grandfathers. I know that I am just as stupid as my own grandfathers were. Therefore I am not about to bow down to an image of God with a white beard!

We intelligent people do not believe in that kind of God, not really. I mean we think that God is spirit, that God is indefinable and infinite and all that sort of thing; but nevertheless, the images of God have a far more powerful effect upon our emotions than on our ideas.

And when people read the Bible and sing hymns like

"Ancient of days who sittest throned in glory" and "Immortal, invisible God only wise, in light inaccessible hid from our eyes," they have still got that fellow up there with a beard. It is way back in the emotions.

To offset this, we should think in contrary imagery, and the contrary imagery is:

> She is black.
> Imagine instead of God the Father,
> God the Mother,
> and instead of an illuminous being blazing with
>   light,
> an unfathomable darkness.

This idea is portrayed in Hindu mythology by Kali, the Great Mother. She is represented in the most terrible imagery. Kali has fangs and a lolling tongue drooling with blood; she has a scimitar in one hand, a severed head in the other, and she is trampling on the body of her husband, Shiva. Shiva represents, furthermore, the destructive aspect of the deity, wherein all things are dissolved so that they can be reborn again. Here is this bloodsucking, terrible mother as the image of the supreme reality behind this universe. She is the representative of all the most awful things of which we are most terrified.

This is a very important image.

Suppose you are presently feeling fairly good. The reason you know you are feeling fairly good is that way far off in the background of your mind, you have got the sensation of something absolutely ghastly that simply must not happen. And so, against that which is not happening and which does not necessarily have to happen, by comparison you feel pretty good.

That absolutely ghastly thing that must not happen is Kali.

We must begin to wonder whether the presence of this Kali is not, in a way, very beneficent. How would you know that things were good unless there were something that was not good at all?

She is black. This is not a final position but a way of beginning to look at a problem and of getting our minds out of their normal ruts.

She, that is to say, the feminine, represents what is philosophically called the negative principle. Of course people in our culture today who support women's liberation do not like to hear the feminine associated with the negative, because the negative has acquired very bad connotations. We say that we should accent the positive; that is a purely male chauvinistic attitude. How would you know if you were outstanding unless by contrast there was something instanding?

You cannot appreciate the convex without the concave. You cannot appreciate the firm without the yielding. Therefore, the so-called negativity of the feminine principle is obviously life-giving and very important.

But we live in a culture that does not notice it. For example, our attention fixes itself upon figures and ignores backgrounds. We see a painting, a representation of a bird, and do not notice the white paper underneath it. We see a printed book and assume what is important and that the page doesn't matter. But if you reconsider the whole thing, how could there be visible printing without the page underlying it?

We somehow consider an underlying position, like the missionary position, to be inferior. But to be underlying is to be *fundamental*.

The word *substance* refers to that which stands underneath (*sub*—underneath and *stance*—stands). To be substantial is to be underlying, to be the support,

the foundation of the world.

This is the great function of the feminine, to be the substance.

The feminine is therefore represented by space, which appears black at night.

Were it not for black and empty space, there would be no possibility whatsoever of seeing the stars. Stars shine out of space and astronomers are beginning to realize that stars are a function of space. Now this seems contrary to our common sense because we think that space is simply nothingness, and do not realize that space is completely basic to everything.

It is like your consciousness. Nobody can imagine what consciousness is. It is the most elusive whatever-it-is of all.

Because it is the background of everything else that we know, we don't really pay much attention to it. We pay attention to the things within the field of consciousness, to the outlines, to the objects, to the so-called things that are in the field of vision, the sounds that are in the field of hearing, and so forth. But what it is—whatever it is—that embraces all of that, we don't pay much attention to it. We cannot even try to think about it.

It is like trying to look at your head. Try to look at your head and what do you find? Not even a black blob in the middle of things; you just do not find anything.

And yet, your head is that out of which you see, just as space is that out of which the stars shine.

There is something very odd about all of this. That which you cannot put your finger on, that which always escapes you, that which is completely elusive—

the blank

—seems to be absolutely necessary for there to be anything whatsoever. Now, let us take this further.

Kali is also the principle of death because she carries a scimitar in one hand and a severed head in the other.

Death is tremendously important to think about. We put it off. Death is swept under the carpet in our culture.

In the hospital they try to keep you alive as long as possible, though it may be an utterly desperate situation. They will not tell you that you are going to die. When relatives have to be informed that it is a "hopeless" case, frequently they are warned not to tell the patient. And all the relatives come around with hollow grins and say, "Well, you'll be all right in about a month, and then we'll go and have a holiday by the sea and listen to the birds." And the dying person knows this is a mockery.

We have made death howl with all kinds of ghouls. We have invented dreadful alternatives. The Christian version of heaven is as abominable as the Christian version of hell. Nobody wants to be in church forever!

Children are absolutely horrified when they hear these hymns which say, "Prostrate before Thy throne to lie and gaze and gaze on Thee." Now, in a very subtle theological way I can wangle the hymn around to make it extremely profound. To be prostrate, and yet to gaze (see) at the same time is *coincidentia oppositorum*, a coincidence of opposites, which is very deep. But to a child it is a crick in the neck.

We are faced with the idea that what might happen after death is that we are going to be confronted by our own judge, the one who knows all about us. This is the Big Papa who knows you were a naughty boy or a naughty girl from the beginning of things. He is going to look right through to the core of your inauthentic existence—and what kind of heebie-jeebies may come up!

Or, you may believe in reincarnation and think that your next life will be the rewards and the punishments for what you have done in this life. You know you got away with murder in this life, and the most awful things are going to happen next time around.

You look upon death as a catastrophe.

Then there are other people who say, "When you're dead, you're dead." Just as though nothing is going to happen at all. So what do you have to worry about? Well, we don't quite like that idea, it spooks us. You know what it would be like to die? To go to sleep and never, never wake up?

There are a lot of things it is not going to be like. It is not going to be like being buried alive. It is not going to be like being in the darkness forever. I tell you, it is going to be as if you never existed at all. Not only you, but everything else as well. There just never was anything, and there is no one to regret it.

And there is no problem.

Think about that for awhile.

It is kind of a weird feeling you get when you really think about that.

Really imagine it.

Just to stop altogether, and you cannot even call it *stop*, because you cannot have stop without start. There was no start, there was just no-thing.

If you think about it, that is the way it was before you were born. If you go back in memories as far as you can go, you get to the same place. And as you go forward in your anticipation of the future, as to what it is going to be like to be dead, then you get funny ideas. That this blankness is the necessary counterpart of what we call *being*.

Now we all think we are alive. We think we are really here. How could we experience that as a reality unless we had once been dead? What gives us any ghost of a notion that we are here except by contrast with the fact that once we were not? And later on, will not be?

This thing is a cycle, like positive and negative poles in electricity. This is the value of the symbolism of

She is black.

She, the womb principle, the receptive, the instanding, the void, and the dark. What could light shine out of except darkness?

If we can grasp this, many fascinating consequences follow.

That there is no true blackness in nature. I have a supposedly black cat, but upon close inspection this cat is dark brown. All shadows are colored. When I feel low sometimes I say, "Help, I'm discolored." Just as there are no black cats, there are not really any black people. I am a somewhat pasty pink rather than a true white, while my so-called black friends are various shades of brown.

At the same time, the use of the word *black* contains something very meaningful. It is the principle of the night. The other side of light is important because it shows us that light cannot be light without black. Therefore, we must abandon the theology in which the light and the darkness are irreconcilably opposed to each other.

It is the most schizophrenic possible view to think of light/white as good, that which is whole and must be preserved, and darkness/black as evil, dirty, and to be abandoned or discarded. The light and the darkness, the white and the black, the yang and the yin, are indispensable to each other.

We do not want to think of the resolution of the two as a kind of muddy mixture of black and white. We try to think what it is that is common to light and darkness, black and white, that escapes our imagination.

When male and female meet—really meet—something happens between them which escapes their imagination.

"I love you."

What does it mean?

A woman may ask a man, "Why do you love me?"

And he fumbles, "I don't know, there is a little something about you that I can't put my finger on. Please don't ask me to explain."

Then on some occasion a man may say, "Oh, the situation is perfectly clear, it's thus and so, everyone understands that," and the woman says, "Well, maybe, but I think there is something you have left out, something very important that you have failed to include in your idea. It doesn't feel right to me."

And this is the everlasting game between the two so that they are interminable mysteries to each other. Women look knowing and think they understand men. And men look fierce and think that they understand women. But it is not so.

Neither understands the other and that is as it should be. If we understood everything completely down to its very roots we would be bored.

Everything would be predictable.

What is more of a bore than knowing a person so well that their reactions to everything under the sun are predictable? You know automatically what their opinions will be on any subject and therefore you do not bother to discuss anything. Indeed, such a predictable person is very vulnerable, because anybody whose habits are completely predictable is, as Don Juan told Carlos Castaneda, easy prey.

Always be surprising and, furthermore, surprise yourself!

The only way that you can be truly irregular is not to know yourself, in your own head, what you are going to do next. This is as Jesus taught. He said that everyone who is born of the Spirit is like the wind which blows where it wills, and you hear its sound but you cannot tell where it is coming from or where it is going. He also advised his disciples that when they were going to speak they were not to think in advance of what they would say, but just wait for the Spirit to give it to them. (Naturally, all clergymen are trained to prepare their sermons carefully in advance!)

It is the unknown that is profoundly scary to most of us.

We fear that God—that is to say, the ground of our being, the energy which we all express—should remain unknown. We fix on all these images of one kind or another, whether it be male or female, light or dark, and we know very well that what is essential to us cannot be gotten at, and that worries us.

To abandon ourselves peacefully and truly in a surrendered way to the possibility of death, to the nonexistence of our memories, of our egos; to flip over from *is*ness to *isnot*ness; to yield to the feminine, which we gladly do when engaged in sexual intercourse, something very closely associated in all symbolic history with death: These are steps that cause us much anxiety.

We are at once fascinated and horrified by this thing that we are that we can never know, never control.

We thus come into the presence of the God who has no image.

Behind the father image, behind the mother image, behind the image of light inaccessible, and behind the image of profound and abysmal darkness, there is something else that we cannot conceive at all. This is not

atheism in the formal sense of the word. It is a profoundly religious attitude, because in practical terms, it
corresponds to an attitude towards life of total trust and
letting go.

When we form images of God they are all really
exhibitions of our lack of faith. We want something to
hold on to, something to grasp, the rock of ages or whatever. But only when we do not grasp, do we have the
attitude of faith.

Ordinarily, if I were to present you with an idea that
seems to you completely negative, abolishing all the
certainties to which you feel you ought to cling and
apparently leaving you in the midst of a void, I would
normally be thought of as a nihilist, a destroyer. It is
true, in a way, that this is a Shiva attitude, a destructive
attitude. But, again, we come to the idea of atheism in
the name of God. Only if you are willing to let go of all
these conceptions can you really discover yourself.

If you let go of all the idols, you will, of course, discover that this unknown which is the foundation of the
universe is precisely you.

> It is not the you you think you are.
> It is not your opinion of yourself.
> It is not your idea or image of yourself.
> It is not your chronic sense of must.
>
> Your self, you see, is way beyond all of that.
> It is something you could never catch hold of.
>
> You cannot grasp it; why would you need to?
> Suppose you could; what would you do with it?
>
> **You can never get at it.**

The attitude of faith towards that profound central mystery is to stop chasing it, grabbing at it.

If that happens, the most amazing things will follow. If I try to improve and control myself by lifting myself up by my own bootstraps, I will waste energy indefinitely; it cannot be done. When I abandon the attempt, suddenly all that energy that I have been wasting is available to something else.

Most of us are in a constant state of tension about whether we are going to survive. Every minute of driving on the freeway you wonder whether you are going to survive. Take an airplane and you wonder whether you are going to survive. You wonder where the money is going to come from to buy groceries tomorrow. We are absolutely absorbed by this need to survive. We are "tired of livin' and scared of dyin'."

Suppose you realize that it does not matter whether you survive. Do you really need to survive?

> Would you not feel much better if you gave up the need to survive?
> Would you not feel free?
> Would you not have more energy available for glorious things?
> Would you not be able to love others more if you were no longer concerned about whether you are going to survive?

We have been taught that we must go on, it is our duty.

It is not.

All these ideas of the spiritual, the godly, and the dutiful are not the only way of being religious.

There is an ineffable mystery that underlies ourselves and the world. It is the darkness from which the light shines. When you recognize the integrity of the universe and that death is as certain as birth, then you can relax and accept that this is the way it is.

There is nothing else to do.

Who Am I?

What is actually going on in the world is far, far different. Every view that we take of the world and every selection we make of what is important to notice is simply one way of looking at things, and there are infinite ways of looking. Considering such things makes us aware of how much our knowledge of the world is conventional knowledge. We attend to a selection of particular things which we have been brainwashed to notice and we disregard the rest. It is as if the world were a Rorschach blot, and there is one official interpretation of the blot, and everybody agrees that is the way it is.

Inevitably, along will come some great genius who will point out that we can look at the world in an entirely different way, and at first everyone will say it is crazy. But if the genius persists long enough, we come to accept the new vision.

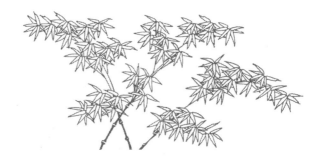

OM: The Sound of Hinduism

OM.

This word is the whole universe.

It is explained that everything
Past
Present and
Future
is the sound OM.

And whatever is beyond these three
    divisions of time
that also, indeed, is OM.

In the beginning
There was only the Self
Like a person alone.
Looking around it saw nothing
Other than itself.

It first said, "I am"
And so there came the name "I."
Thus, to this day
When one is asked, "Who is there?"
He replies, "It is I," and then
Gives what other name he may have.

The Self was afraid, as
One who is alone is afraid.
But it thought
Since there is nothing beside my self
Of what am I afraid?

Whereat the fear vanished.

For what could it have feared?
Fear can only come from something other.

But the Self had no delight
As one alone has no delight.
It desired another.
It expanded to the form of male and female
    in tight embrace.
And then fell into two parts.
Thus it is that everybody is one half
Like one of the halves of a split pea.
And the missing half is filled by a spouse.

Then he coupled with her
And produced all human beings.
She thought,
"How can he have intercourse with me
having produced me from himself?
I will hide."

She became a cow.
But he became a bull, and
Coupling with her,
produced all cattle.

And, in turn, she became
A mare, and he, a stallion.

She, a female donkey, and
He, a male donkey.

She, a she-goat, and
He, a he-goat.

She, a ewe, and
He, a ram.

And Thus were born
from their union
All beings that exist in pairs
Down to the very ants.

He knew.
I am, in fact, this universe
For I have produced it all.

In this way, he became the universe.

There was never a time when I was not,
Nor you, nor these others.
Nor will there ever be a time to come
When we shall cease.

As one passes in this body
Through childhood, youth, and old age
Even so is the taking on of other bodies.

This does not trouble the wise.

Of the nonexistent
There is no coming to be.
Of the existent
There is no ceasing to be.

That by which all this is pervaded
Cannot be destroyed.

As one casts off wornout clothes
And puts on others that are new
Even so the Self casts off wornout bodies
And assumes others that are new.

Weapons cannot cut this Self
Fire cannot burn it
Water does not make it wet
Nor the wind, dry.

It is eternal
All-pervading
Changeless and
Unmoved.

It is the same forever
It is said to be unmanifest
Inconceivable, and
Without change.

Knowing it thus
You should not breathe.

The Knower
The central Self
Is not born
And does not die.

It is not produced from anything
And produces nothing apart from itself.
It is unborn, eternal, enduring, primordial.
It is not slain when the body is slain.
If the slayer thinks he slays
Or the slain thinks he is slain
Neither understands
It neither slays nor can be slain.

Smaller than the small
Greater than the great
It is the self in the heart of all being.

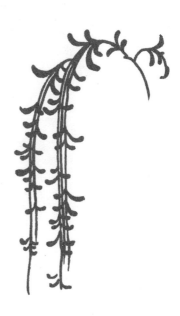

By whose direction is the mind aware
    of objects?

By whose command does life first move?

By whose will is this speaking uttered?

And what god empowers the eye and
    the ear?

It is the hearing of the ear
The awareness of the mind
The very sound of speech
The life of the breath
And the sight of the eye.

Therefore the wise,
Surrendering themselves,
Go beyond this world
And are immortal.

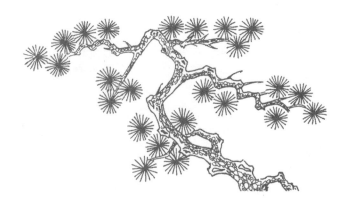

But IT is beyond the reach of sight, speech,
    and thought
And we neither know nor understand
How it can be taught.

IT is other than the known
And beyond the unknown
Thus we have heard from the wise.

IT is that which cannot be spoken
But by which we speak.

IT is that which cannot be thought
But by which we think.

IT is that which cannot be seen
But by which we see.

IT is that which cannot be heard
But by which we hear.

IT is the breath which cannot be held
But by which we breathe.

IT is known to those who do not know;
To those who know it, it is unknown.

IT is not understood by those who
    understand it;
IT is understood by those who
    understand it not.

Listen.
Listen down.
Down to that sound.
What is it?
A current of air?
Vibrating vocal cords?
Your own eardrums?
Something running in your head?
It's all of these.
This sound is you vibrating.
This sound is you.

And who are you?

Don't give me your name, address,
    and occupation.
You know that's just a mask, a front,
    a Big Act.
Who puts it on? Your body?
What an act that is!
And who puts that on?
Your father and mother. Did they
    put you on?
Come off it.

You know very well who you are,
    but you won't admit it.
Deep in there in the middle,
    middle of your heart you know it.
You've always been around and
    always will be.

And the you in you is the same as
    the you in me.

You're not some tourist just visiting in
    this world for a short time.
You belong here, like the apple on the tree.
And, as the apple is the energy of the tree,
you...yes, you...are the energy of the world.

You don't know who you are, do you?
You can't really get at yourself.
Just as the fingertip can't touch itself and
the teeth can't bite themselves.

And that's because you,
The far-in you,
Is what we call Brahman.
The Self of the universe.
The *which* of which there is no *whicher*.
The heart and foundation of all that's
    going on.

You think you're going to die someday. Yes.
That's because every now and then
You have to go *Off*
So that you can know you are *On*.
You can't have an up without a down,
A back without a front,
A light day without a dark night.
The whole thing is pulse.

So what are you doing, Brahman?
You're playing *On* and *Off* with yourself,
Hide and seek with yourself.
You're just passing eternal time
     with adventure.
You forget who you are, really.

Every now and then you pretend you're
     just a
John Doe, or a
Mary Smith, or a
Butterfly, or a
Worm, or a
Star.
And that you are lost in the middle of
     a big, big Outside World.
That isn't you.
That you don't understand.
That you don't control.

Of course,
There has to be something Other
To bring out the feeling that
You are you.
And, so that you can feel really you,
That outside world has to feel really
Strange, different, weird.

You old trickster!

Deep down in
You know the whole bit and
What you want is surprise.
So you have to let things get out of control.
You have to feel lost and lonely
To know you are you.
And you play the thing out
By inventing lusts and loves
Fears and terror
Gnawing anxieties and
Screaming meemies.

All so you can imagine it's not really *you*
It is IT
That runs the show.

But our secret is...

You are IT!

You are running the show.
By not letting your right-hand know what
    your left-hand is doing.
By making life a whopping great
    split between
What you do and
What happens to you.
This is the great illusion, the play,
The Big Act.

And you don't just play your game
With such simple elements as
On and Off
Black and white
Life and death.

To seem as real as real can be
This world that you are playing must be
So complicated that you can't figure it out.

So between
Black and white
There is the whole range of colors.

Between a smashing fist in the face and
Trying to touch the air
There are all the textures of
Feeling
Burning
Throbbing
Pushing
Hugging
Fondling
Tickling
Kissing
Brushing
and light wind on the skin.

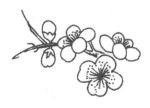

Your world is all these elements
Of life and sound
Of taste, smell, and touch
Woven together in many dimensions on the
Fabulous loom of your brain.

Your brain.
The most complicated thing in the world.
Which you yourself grew without even
    thinking about it.

You have always been you
For you, I, the Self
Is simply what there is and
All that there is.
All of us are rays from one center,
Tits on one sow,
Sounds on one flute.
Forever and ever.

But it doesn't get monotonous
Or boring
Because we keep forgetting it.

We keep the *Ons* on
By putting *Offs* between them.

How big is IT?
How long is On?
How long is Off?

Say that man and woman, human life,
Is a dance that lasts 4,320,000 years.
(Just to give an idea of the vastness.)
And of course
There are all sorts of other dances going on
    at the same time
With their own rhythms.
Star dances
Rock dances
Fish dances
Insect dances
Plant dances
And strange animal scenes like
Crocodile dances
Elephant dances.

The human dance runs for 4,320,000 years,
A span of time that we call a kalpa.
Before it begins and
After it ends
There is always another kalpa
Or off-period
During which the self is simply the self
And doesn't pretend to be this me or
    that you.
We call this rest period
Peace. Uninvolvement. Pure bliss.

When the 4,320,000 years of rest crawl to
    a close
The dance begins again
Although it always seems like the
    first time.
Every day is today.

And then
Through many centuries
Through many pulses of waking and
    sleeping
Life and death
You stretch your world out through a span
    of time that
Varies in mood
Like a rainbow, running from
Purple to red, from
Royal delight to destruction and fire. For
As there is no purple without red
There is no pleasure without pain.

There are four great divisions of the kalpa.
They have been likened to the four throws
    in the Hindu game of dice.
First is the perfect throw of four.
Next, the slightly imperfect throw of three.
Then, the throw of two, and
Finally, the worst throw of one.

And so the first period runs for
    1,728,000 years
During which the whole world is as perfect
as a fresh flower and
as unblemished as the skin of a young girl.

The second period is a little shorter.
It runs for 1,296,000 years
During which a small element of evil and
    decay comes into life
And the tips of the petals are very
    slightly brown.

The third period runs for 864,000 years.
In this age the powers of evil and good are
    evenly balanced.

The fourth period runs for only
    432,000 years
In which the powers of evil and destruction
    take over.

At the end
Your eternal Self
Takes the form of Shiva, the lord of renewal
    through death
Blue-bodied and ten-armed with a necklace
    of skulls.
But with one hand in a gesture that
    reminds us that all this is
Illusion and play.
The Shiva dances the dance of fire
In which the material world is destroyed.
And the Self returns to the state of
Peace
Uninvolvement and
Pure bliss.

All of this goes on forever
Through kalpa after kalpa after kalpa,
And not only in this visible world
That we call the universe.

For this universe that we know
Is only a speck of dust in another universe,
And all the specks of dust in this universe
    that we know
Contain minute universes without measure.
Boundless inward in the atom.
Boundless outward in the cold.
However vast
However incomprehensible
However terrifying this entire display may
    seem to be
All of it is at root
Your own innermost Self
The self that you cannot touch
Or see
Or pin down
Or control
Because it is too close
Too near
Right in the middle of everything.

Because it is you.

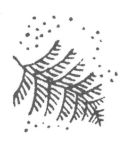

Who Am I?

Now obviously there is a way in which you can see the world for yourself; it may very well agree with what other people see and you will be able to communicate that way of seeing to others. It may be by no more than a glint in the eye that you will know someone else sees it just as you do.

All our meditation practices are simply to open our consciousness to what is going on, as distinct from what is "said" to be going on. To do that, we must suspend our words, suspend our descriptions, and be alert to the actual happening. It is as simple as that.

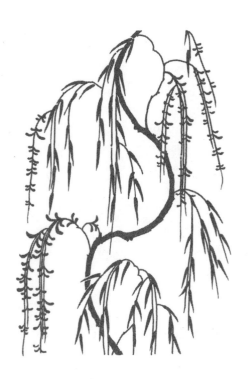

DYANA II: A *Guided Meditation*

M editation has no purpose or objective except to be entirely here and now. It is not something you do to improve yourself, to get ahead in the world, or to prepare yourself for life. For the division of time into past, present, and future is a trick of words and numbers. All memories and expectations exist now and now only, because now is what there is and all that there is. We could say that the past flows back from now like the wake from the prow of a ship, and then, just like the wake, vanishes. As the wake does not drive the ship, the past does not propel or move the present unless you, here and now, want to insist that it does, and so give yourself a perpetual alibi for every kind of irresponsibility. But I am not preaching; that would be a diversion from our feeling-center, this eternal here and now.

So then, we are going to try to find out and feel what we mean by "now." Is now a split second, or is it a drawn out expanse of sensation? Try this. Just stand up for a moment and take three steps forward, one, two, three, and stop. Where, at this moment, is the first step you took? And where is the next movement you are going to make? Hold it. Be still. The next movement hasn't happened. Past movements aren't here. Where are you? When are you? What is the position of the universe? When is it? Where is it? Take another step. Is this a new now or the same old now where you always were? The next step is not with your feet, but with your imagination. Recall the first step that you just made. Now when are you? Back then or still here? So please sit down again and relax.

For meditation, it is best to sit on the floor or on a cushion, spine straight, hands with palms upward resting upon each other. The reason for this position is that it is firm and grounded and just uncomfortable enough to keep you from going to sleep, but do not fight the discomfort. Relax into the position, just as you have learned how to relax and to ease out a long, long breath, and so create energy without strain.

In the same way, if you have understood that there is no time but now, you will be able, without the least difficulty, to sit in this way for a long time as measured by the clock. Will you try an experiment with me? Simply allow your ears to hear all sounds around you. Just let all sounds going on play upon your eardrums without trying to name, identify, or locate them. Relax your tongue, and let it just float in your lower jaw. Close your eyes for a moment.

If you are still thinking in words, or calculating about this, that, and the other that you are supposed to be doing, do not try to stop it. Just let your mind do whatever it likes, and hear its chatter as if you were listening to rippling water. Do not try to name or identify these sounds. Just hear them as you would listen to music, as when you hear a flute, or a guitar without asking what it means. Do not bother about what it means. Your brain will take care of that by itself. Just let your eardrums respond as they will to all vibrations now in the air. Do not let yourself, or your ears, be offended by improper or unscheduled sounds. If, for example, a recording is scratchy, it is okay. You would not object to it if you were listening to it sitting by a fire of crackling logs. It is just a noise. Keep your tongue relaxed, floating easily in the lower jaw. Also, stop frowning. Allow the space between your eyes to feel easy and open, and just let the vibrations in the air play with your ears.

In meditation we are concerned only with what is; with reality—nothing else. The past is a memory; the future, an expectation. Neither past nor future actually exists. There is simply eternal now. So do not seek or expect a result from what you do. That would not be true meditation. There is no hurry. Just know you are not going anywhere. Simply be here. Live in the world of sound. In the world of pure sound, can you actually hear anyone who is listening? Can you hear any difference between all these sounds, on the one hand, and yourself, on the other? Naturally, we use techniques and gimmicks to help the thinking mind to become silent and one of them is the gong. It is a sound at once pleasing and compelling. It absorbs tension, and when it fades out, the one sound becomes the many. The single tone is transformed easily and gently into all other noises. And that is how the universe comes into being, out of the one energy underlying all events.

If you do not have a gong, you can use your own voice

by chanting what Hindus and Buddhists call a *mantram*, and that is a syllable or phrase sung for its sound, rather than its meaning. Chief of these is the syllable *om*, spelled phonetically "a-u-m." It is called the *pranava* or the sound of God, because it involves the whole range of the voice from the back of the throat to the lips. Take the tone from the back of the throat to your lips. You can hear all sounds as "Om." They are all at some point in the total range of sound from the back of the throat to the lips, making a spectrum of sound, as all colors are originally one white light. But do not ask what the sound is or what it means; just hear it and dig it.

Let me explain again what we are doing. We are going behind words, names, numbers, beliefs, and ideas to get back to the naked experience of reality itself and, at this level of awareness, we find no difference between the listener and the sound, the knower and the known, the subject and the object, or between the past, the present, and the future. All that is just talk. What is really happening is right now. Chanting and meditation depends on the regulation of the breath in a way which is basic to the art of meditation and I am going to show you how to do this and why. To begin with, just as you have been letting vibrations in the air play with your ears, let your lungs breathe as they will. Do not, as yet, attempt any breathing exercise, do not force anything. Simply allow breathing. Now is this breathing a voluntary or involuntary action, or both, or neither? Just feel it without taking sides, without words. Hear your voice as if it were wind in the trees or the sound of waves.

Most of us are short of breath. We never really empty

our lungs. To make a long, complete outbreath, you must not force it. Imagine there is a large ball of lead inside your neck and allow it to fall slowly through your body to the floor, pushing, and easing the breath out as it drops. Ease the breath out just as you settle and sink down comfortably into a bed. When the ball reaches the floor, let it drop away as if to the center of the earth. Then let the breath come back in as a reflex without pulling it. And then imagine another ball of lead in the neck and, again, let it fall out, long and easy.

And once again.

And now, do you see what is happening? You are generating a great deal of energy without trying or forcing. Two things seem to be happening at once: First, the outflow of breath is simply falling, happening all by itself. Second, it is under perfect control. So, from this practice, you learn to experience, to realize that what happens to you, and what you do, are one and the same process. There is no real separation between one thing called "you" and another quite different thing called "the universe." When you stop talking and naming, they are quite obviously one. So again, let your breath fall easily out. All the way. Let it come back on its own, and then out again.

And now, let us put the sound "Om" on the next outflow.

And again, so that you have nothing in mind but "Om."

Once again, the essence of the whole art is to feel, to experience, to sense what is, what happens, without defining it, without saying anything to yourself about it.

So, let your breath flow easily, heavily, down and out again with no strain.

And after it has come back in, once more.

Keep it up. Well then, who are you? What are you? What am I? Some people say, it is this body. Others say the mind, the ego, or the soul. But all those, including the body, are names and notions. Can we experience the self directly like a sound, a flame, or any other object? Put your hands on that mysteriously invisible thing known as your head. Keep your eyes open, blinking occasionally without staring. Let us assume that all ordinary ideas of what I am are either so wrong or so doubtful that we must investigate the matter directly. However, to do that you must first get the sensation or the feeling of yourself without forming any idea. Regard words in the head as mere noise. Just stop, look, and listen.

Now, let the various colors and shapes before you play with your eyes, just as you have been letting sounds play with your ears. Where are they—out in front of your face, or inside your brain in the optical nervous system? Is your head in the world or is the world in your head, or both? Odd, isn't it? Either you were everything you felt, or you just did not feel yourself, the feeler, at all, just as you did not see your eyes. All or nothing. As is said in an ancient Chinese text called the *Secret of the Golden Flower*, between the all and the void is only a difference of name.

Now, put your hands back on your lap, palms upward, one upon the other, and just let go of it all. Let your ears hear whatever they like. Let the nerve ends in your skin feel whatever they like. Let your eyes see whatever they like. Let your nose smell whatever it likes. Let your mind think whatever it likes. Let your lungs breathe as they will. And let things happen as they happen. Are these all different senses or just one sense?

The sound of the rain needs no translation, no explanation.

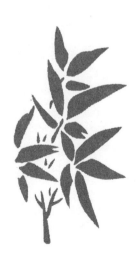

Alan Watts Audio Collection

ORIGINAL LIVE RECORDINGS FROM
ELECTRONIC UNIVERSITY

The Tao of Philosophy—Volume I

❏ *Slices of Wisdom*—Notable segments drawn from the first thirteen weeks of the "Love of Wisdom" public radio series. (29 min.)

❏ *Images of God*—Watts explores the metaphysics underlying feminine symbolism in images of the divine throughout the world, in which "the deep" and "the dark" are recognized as the unifying ground of being. (29 min.)

❏ *Sense of Nonsense*—Recorded live on KPFA, this popular program is a delightful excursion into the essential purposelessness of life. (29 min.)

❏ *Coincidence of Opposites*—Just as the purpose of dancing is not to arrive at a certain place on the floor, life has no concrete goal to be achieved. (29 min.)

❏ *Seeing Through the Net*—In a sparkling 1969 talk to IBM systems engineers, Watts describes the "net" of perception we throw over reality, and the contrasting perceptions of "prickles" and "goo." (58 min.)

❏ *Myth of Myself*—What do we mean when we use the word "I"? Could self-image be the barrier to knowing who and what we really are? (42 min.)

❏ *Man and Nature*—Western culture sees the world as a mechanical system while Eastern philosophies see it as an all-encompassing organic process. Just as an apple tree "apples," the earth "peoples," and we are not so much born into this world as grown out of it. (56 min.)

❏ *Symbols and Meaning*—As symbols, words point to things they represent, and thus have meaning. By contrast, life itself does not stand for anything else, and therefore has no meaning in the usual sense. (29 min.)

❏ *Limits of Language*—Watts suggests that language may alter our view of reality, and by knowing the limits of language we can move on to the unspeakable. (29 min.)

The Philosophies of Asia—Volume I

❏ *Relevance of Oriental Philosophy*—Alan Watts looks at Eastern thought in contrast with the religions of the Western world. Chinese and Indian models are used to point out how we can better understand our own culture by contrasting it with others. (56 min.)

❏ *Mythology of Hinduism*—An engaging overview of the Hindu perspective on the universe, its theory of time and the concept of an underlying godhead which is dreaming all of us. (54 min.)

❏ *EcoZen*—Speaking before a college audience, Watts points out that "ecological awareness" and "mystical experience" are different ways of saying the same thing. (29 min.)

❏ *A Ball of Hot Iron*—Continuing an introduction toward the understanding of Zen Buddhism, Watts describes the essential unity of the organism and its environment. (29 min.)

The Philosophies of Asia—Volume II

❏ *Intellectual Yoga*—In a lively discussion of the intellect as a path to one's enlightenment, Watts overseas that "it is amazing how many things there are that aren't so." (42 min.)

❏ *Introduction to Buddhism*—Buddhism is traced from its origins in India to China, and then on to Japan. Along the way Watts brings to life one of the world's great religious traditions in its many forms, from the Theravada school to contemporary Zen. (58 min.)

❏ *Taoist Way of Karma I*—The word karma literally means "doing" and is thus "your doing" or action. Taoism suggests a spontaneous course of action in accord with the current and grain of nature. (29 min.)

❏ *Taoist Way of Karma II*—By following the Tao or course of nature, one comes into harmony with the world and drops out of the cycles of karma perpetuated by our attempts to control destiny. (29 min.)

Each of the preceding volumes consists of three audio cassettes in an attractive bookshelf binder. The price for each volume is $29.95. To order by phone, call (800) 969-2887. To order by mail, write to the address on the following page. Please add $3 per item for shipping.

Also Available

❏ **EASTERN AND WESTERN ZEN**—*Zen Stories* (50 min.); *Uncarved Block, Unbleached Silk* (44 min.); *Biting the Iron Bull* (45 min.); *Swimming Headless* (51 min.); *Wisdom on the Ridiculous* (46 min.); *Zen Bones* (59 min.)

❏ **BUDDHISM**—*The Journey from India* (40 min.); *Following the Middle Way* (42 min.); *Buddhism as Dialogue* (62 min.); *The Importance of Folly* (58 min.); *Transcending Duality* (47 min.); *The Diamond Web* (40 min.)

❏ **PHILOSOPHY AND SOCIETY**—*On Time and Death* (50 min.); *The Cosmic Drama* (45 min.); *Philosophy of Nature* (45 min.); *What is Reality?* (50 min.); *Mysticism and Morals* (58 min.); *On Being God* (60 min.)

❏ **MYTH AND RELIGION**—*Not What Should Be* (60 min.); *Spiritual Authority* (55 min.); *Jesus—His Religion or the Religion About Him?* (56 min.); *Democracy in the Kingdom of Heaven* (50 min.); *The Image of Man* (50 min.); *Sex in the Church* (52 min.)

Each of the six-cassette audio series above has its own attractive bookshelf binder. The regular list price for each series is $59.95. However, you may select any two series for $100, any three for $140, or all four for $175.

Please add $3 for priority mail per set, $10 per set for overnight mail, or $5 per set for overseas shipping. We accept Visa, MasterCard, and American Express cards.

ELECTRONIC UNIVERSITY
P.O. Box 2309, San Anselmo, CA 94979
(800) 969-2887

Also Available from Celestial Arts

The Essential Alan Watts by Alan Watts

Revised by his son Mark, we have the last original work
of Alan Watts now combined with several favorite pieces
previously unavailable in book form (including the classics
Work as Play and *The Trickster Guru*). Also included are *Ego*;
Time; *The More Things Change*; *The Drama of It All*; *Oriental
"Omnipotence"*; *Psychotherapy and Eastern Religion*; *The
Individual as Man/World*; and *Speaking Personally*

156 pages, 5½ x 8½, quality paperback

The Early Writings of Alan Watts
Edited by John Snelling with Mark Watts

This first volume of the early writings of Alan Watts covers
the period from 1931, when he was still a schoolboy, to
1938, when he departed from Britain for the United States.
This book includes all the earliest published pieces by Alan
Watts—many essays, book reviews, poems, and letters—
showing in chronological order the early development of
Watts' thought.

Since 1980, John Snelling has served as the editor of
The Middle Way.

288 pages, 5½ x 8½, quality paperback

Available at your local bookstore or order direct from the
publisher. For ordering information call (800) 841-2665.

CELESTIAL ARTS • P.O. Box 7123, Berkeley, CA 94707.